Maritza Montero, PhD
Editor

Leadership and Organization for Community Prevention and Intervention in Venezuela

Leadership and Organization for Community Prevention and Intervention in Venezuela has been co-published simultaneously as *Journal of Prevention & Intervention in the Community*, Volume 27, Number 1 2004.

Pre-publication
REVIEWS,
COMMENTARIES,
EVALUATIONS . . .

"INTERESTING. . . . OF WIDE RELEVANCE TO ALL COMMUNITY PSYCHOLOGISTS who work with community systems and especially with disadvantaged communities. The book provides a taxonomy of types of community leadership, develops the idea of 'metadecision,' and identifies complex characteristics of family and community interaction patterns in the disadvantaged barrios of Caracas. The authors consider the relationships among community leaders, social organization in poor communities, participation in community development, struggle, and change. As such, a fascinating insight is provided into social and community life that, while based in the particular situation of Venezuelan low-income neighborhoods, has a wider relevance to how we can understand the life and organization of any community."

Mark Burton, PhD, MSc, AFBPS
Head, Manchester Learning Disability Partnership
Visiting Professor
University of Northubria at Newcastle
Member, Community and Organisational Psychology Research Group
Manchester Metropolitan University

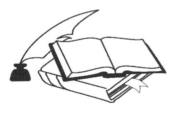

"This book opens a window onto the complex social struggles taking place in contemporary Venezuela, and PROVIDES A FASCINATING INSIGHT INTO THE DIFFICULT PROCESS OF NEGOTIATING NEW FORMS OF COMMUNITY LEADERSHIP. Maritza Montero is one of the leading radical forces in community psychology in Latin America, and she brings her keen grasp of the politics of local communities to bear on the most urgent issues facing the Venezuelan people. Montero has gathered together an impressive range of academics and community activists, and THE BOOK IS TESTIMONY TO WHAT CAN BE DONE INSIDE THE DOMINANT INSTITUTIONS to bring them face-to-face with forces of resistance and change in the real world."

Ian Parker, PhD
Professor of Psychology
Manchester Metropolitan University
United Kingdom

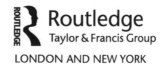

Routledge
Taylor & Francis Group

LONDON AND NEW YORK

Leadership and Organization for Community Prevention and Intervention in Venezuela

Leadership and Organization for Community Prevention and Intervention in Venezuela has been co-published simultaneously as *Journal of Prevention & Intervention in the Community*, Volume 27, Number 1 2004.

The *Journal of Prevention & Intervention in the Community*™ Monographic "Separates" (formerly the *Prevention in Human Services* series)*

For information on previous issues of *Prevention in Human Services*, edited by Robert E. Hess, please contact: The Haworth Press, Inc., 10 Alice Street, Binghamton, NY 13904-1580 USA.

Below is a list of "separates," which in serials librarianship means a special issue simultaneously published as a special journal issue or double-issue *and* as a "separate" hardbound monograph. (This is a format which we also call a "DocuSerial.")

"Separates" are published because specialized libraries or professionals may wish to purchase a specific thematic issue by itself in a format which can be separately cataloged and shelved, as opposed to purchasing the journal on an on-going basis. Faculty members may also more easily consider a "separate" for classroom adoption.

"Separates" are carefully classified separately with the major book jobbers so that the journal tie-in can be noted on new book order slips to avoid duplicate purchasing.

You may wish to visit Haworth's website at . . .

http://www.HaworthPress.com

. . . to search our online catalog for complete tables of contents of these separates and related publications.

You may also call 1-800-HAWORTH (outside US/Canada: 607-722-5857), or Fax 1-800-895-0582 (outside US/Canada: 607-771-0012), or e-mail at:

docdelivery@haworthpress.com

Leadership and Organization for Community Prevention and Intervention in Venezuela, edited by Maritza Montero, PhD (Vol. 27, No. 1, 2004). *Shows how (and why) participatory communities come into being, what they can accomplish, and how to help their leaders develop the skills they need to be most effective.*

Empowerment and Participatory Evaluation of Community Interventions: Multiple Benefits, edited by Yolanda Suarez-Balcazar, PhD, and Gary W. Harper, PhD, MPH (Vol. 26, No. 2, 2003). *"USEFUL. . . . Draws together diverse chapters that uncover the how and why of empowerment and participatory evaluation while offering exemplary case studies showing the challenges and successes of this community value-based evaluation model."* (Anne E. Brodsky, PhD, Associate Professor of Psychology, University of Maryland Baltimore County)

Traumatic Stress and Its Aftermath: Cultural, Community, and Professional Contexts, edited by Sandra S. Lee, PhD (Vol. 26, No. 1, 2003). *Explores risk and protective factors for traumatic stress, emphasizing the impact of cumulative/multiple trauma in a variety of populations, including therapists themselves.*

Culture, Peers, and Delinquency, edited by Clifford O'Donnell, PhD (Vol. 25, No. 2, 2003). *"TIMELY . . . . OF VALUE TO BOTH STUDENTS AND PROFESSIONALS. . . . Demonstrates how peers can serve as a pathway to delinquency from a multiethnic perspective. The discussion of ethnic, racial, and gender differences challenges the field to reconsider assessment, treatment, and preventative approaches."* (Donald Meichenbaum, PhD, Distinguished Professor Emeritus, University of Waterloo, Ontario, Canada; Research Director, The Melissa Institute for Violence Prevention and the Treatment of Victims of Violence, Miami, Florida)

Prevention and Intervention Practice in Post-Apartheid South Africa, edited by Vijé Franchi, PhD, and Norman Duncan, PhD, consulting editor (Vol. 25, No.1, 2003). *"Highlights the way in which preventive and curative interventions serve–or do not serve–the ideals of equality, empowerment, and participation. . . . Revolutionizes our way of thinking about and teaching socio-pedagogical action in the context of exclusion."* (Dr. Altay A. Manço, Scientific Director, Institute of Research, Training, and Action on Migrations, Belgium)

Community Interventions to Create Change in Children, edited by Lorna H. London, PhD (Vol. 24, No. 2, 2002). *"Illustrates creative approaches to prevention and intervention with at-risk youth. . . . Describes multiple methods to consider in the design, implementation, and evaluation of pro - grams."* (Susan D. McMahon, PhD, Assistant Professor, Department of Psychology, DePaul University)

Preventing Youth Access to Tobacco, edited by Leonard A. Jason, PhD, and Steven B. Pokorny, PhD (Vol. 24, No. 1, 2002). *"Explores cutting-edge issues in youth access research methodology .... Provides a thorough review of the tobacco control literature and detailed analysis of the methodological issues presented by community interventions to increase the effectiveness of tobacco control. . . . Challenges widespread assumptions about the dynamics of youth access programs and the requirements for long-term success."* (John A. Gardiner, PhD, LLB, Consultant to the 2000 Surgeon General's Report Reducing Youth Access to Tobacco and to the National Cancer Institute's evaluation of the ASSIST program)

The Transition from Welfare to Work: Processes, Challenges, and Outcomes, edited by Sharon Telleen, PhD, and Judith V. Sayad (Vol. 23, No. 1/2, 2002). *A comprehensive examination of the welfare-to-work initiatives surrounding the major reform of United States welfare legislation in 1996.*

Prevention Issues for Women's Health in the New Millennium, edited by Wendee M. Wechsberg, PhD (Vol. 22, No. 2, 2001). *"Helpful to service providers as well as researchers ... A useful ancillary textbook for courses addressing women's health issues. Covers a wide range of health issues affecting women."* (Sherry Deren, PhD, Director, Center for Drug Use and HIV Research, National Drug Research Institute, New York City)

Workplace Safety: Individual Differences in Behavior, edited by Alice F. Stuhlmacher, PhD, and Douglas F. Cellar, PhD (Vol. 22, No. 1, 2001). Workplace Safety: Individual Differences in Behavior *examines safety behavior and outlines practical interventions to help increase safety awareness. Individual differences are relevant to a variety of settings, including the workplace, public spaces, and motor vehicles. This book takes a look at ways of defining and measuring safety as well as a variety of individual differences like gender, job knowledge, conscientiousness, self-efficacy, risk avoidance, and stress tolerance that are important in creating safety interventions and improving the selection and training of employees.* Workplace Safety *takes an incisive look at these issues with a unique focus on the way individual differences in people impact safety behavior in the real world.*

People with Disabilities: Empowerment and Community Action, edited by Christopher B. Keys, PhD, and Peter W. Dowrick, PhD (Vol. 21, No. 2, 2001). *"Timely and useful ... provides valuable lessons and guidance for everyone involved in the disability movement. This book is a must-read for researchers and practitioners interested in disability rights issues!"* (Karen M. Ward, EdD, Director, Center for Human Development; Associate Professor, University of Alaska, Anchorage)

Family Systems/Family Therapy: Applications for Clinical Practice, edited by Joan D. Atwood, PhD (Vol. 21, No. 1, 2001). *Examines family therapy issues in the context of the larger systems of health, law, and education and suggests ways family therapists can effectively use an intersystems approach.*

HIV/AIDS Prevention: Current Issues in Community Practice, edited by Doreen D. Salina, PhD (Vol. 19, No. 1, 2000). *Helps researchers and psychologists explore specific methods of improving HIV/AIDS prevention research.*

Educating Students to Make-a-Difference: Community-Based Service Learning, edited by Joseph R. Ferrari, PhD, and Judith G. Chapman, PhD (Vol. 18, No. 1/2, 1999). *"There is something here for everyone interested in the social psychology of service-learning."* (Frank Bernt, PhD, Associate Professor, St. Joseph's University)

Program Implementation in Preventive Trials, edited by Joseph A. Durlak and Joseph R. Ferrari, PhD (Vol. 17, No. 2, 1998). *"Fills an important gap in preventive research. . . . Highlights an array of important questions related to implementation and demonstrates just how good community-based intervention programs can be when issues related to implementation are taken seriously."* (Judy Primavera, PhD, Associate Professor of Psychology, Fairfield University, Fairfield, Connecticut)

Preventing Drunk Driving, edited by Elsie R. Shore, PhD, and Joseph R. Ferrari, PhD (Vol. 17, No. 1, 1998). *"A must read for anyone interested in reducing the needless injuries and death caused by the drunk driver."* (Terrance D. Schiavone, President, National Commission Against Drunk Driving, Washington, DC)

Manhood Development in Urban African-American Communities, edited by Roderick J. Watts, PhD, and Robert J. Jagers (Vol. 16, No. 1/2, 1998). *"Watts and Jagers provide the much-needed foundational and baseline information and research that begins to philosophically and empirically validate the importance of understanding culture, oppression, and gender when working with males in urban African-American communities." (Paul Hill, Jr., MSW, LISW, ACSW, East End Neighborhood House, Cleveland, Ohio)*

Diversity Within the Homeless Population: Implications for Intervention, edited by Elizabeth M. Smith, PhD, and Joseph R. Ferrari, PhD (Vol. 15, No. 2, 1997). *"Examines why homelessness is increasing, as well as treatment options, case management techniques, and community intervention programs that can be used to prevent homelessness." (American Public Welfare Association)*

Education in Community Psychology: Models for Graduate and Undergraduate Programs, edited by Clifford R. O'Donnell, PhD, and Joseph R. Ferrari, PhD (Vol. 15, No. 1, 1997). *"An invaluable resource for students seeking graduate training in community psychology . . . [and will] also serve faculty who want to improve undergraduate teaching and graduate programs." (Marybeth Shinn, PhD, Professor of Psychology and Coordinator, Community Doctoral Program, New York University, New York, New York)*

Adolescent Health Care: Program Designs and Services, edited by John S. Wodarski, PhD, Marvin D. Feit, PhD, and Joseph R. Ferrari, PhD (Vol. 14, No. 1/2, 1997). *Devoted to helping practitioners address the problems of our adolescents through the use of preventive interventions based on sound empirical data.*

Preventing Illness Among People with Coronary Heart Disease, edited by John D. Piette, PhD, Robert M. Kaplan, PhD, and Joseph R. Ferrari, PhD (Vol. 13, No. 1/2, 1996). *"A useful contribution to the interaction of physical health, mental health, and the behavioral interventions for patients with CHD." (Public Health: The Journal of the Society of Public Health)*

Sexual Assault and Abuse: Sociocultural Context of Prevention, edited by Carolyn F. Swift, PhD* (Vol. 12, No. 2, 1995). *"Delivers a cornucopia for all who are concerned with the primary prevention of these damaging and degrading acts." (George J. McCall, PhD, Professor of Sociology and Public Administration, University of Missouri)*

International Approaches to Prevention in Mental Health and Human Services, edited by Robert E. Hess, PhD, and Wolfgang Stark* (Vol. 12, No. 1, 1995). *Increases knowledge of prevention strategies from around the world.*

Self-Help and Mutual Aid Groups: International and Multicultural Perspectives, edited by Francine Lavoie, PhD, Thomasina Borkman, PhD, and Benjamin Gidron* (Vol. 11, No. 1/2, 1995). *"A helpful orientation and overview, as well as useful data and methodological suggestions." (International Journal of Group Psychotherapy)*

Prevention and School Transitions, edited by Leonard A. Jason, PhD, Karen E. Danner, and Karen S. Kurasaki, MA* (Vol. 10, No. 2, 1994). *"A collection of studies by leading ecological and systems-oriented theorists in the area of school transitions, describing the stressors, personal resources available, and coping strategies among different groups of children and adolescents undergoing school transitions." (Reference & Research Book News)*

Religion and Prevention in Mental Health: Research, Vision, and Action, edited by Kenneth I. Pargament, PhD, Kenneth I. Maton, PhD, and Robert E. Hess, PhD* (Vol. 9, No. 2 & Vol. 10, No. 1, 1992). *"The authors provide an admirable framework for considering the important, yet often overlooked, differences in theological perspectives." (Family Relations)*

Families as Nurturing Systems: Support Across the Life Span, edited by Donald G. Unger, PhD, and Douglas R. Powell, PhD* (Vol. 9, No. 1, 1991). *"A useful book for anyone thinking about alternative ways of delivering a mental health service." (British Journal of Psychiatry)*

Ethical Implications of Primary Prevention, edited by Gloria B. Levin, PhD, and Edison J. Trickett, PhD* (Vol. 8, No. 2, 1991). *"A thoughtful and thought-provoking summary of ethical issues related to intervention programs and community research." (Betty Tableman, MPA, Director, Division. of Prevention Services and Demonstration Projects, Michigan Department of Mental Health, Lansing)*

Monographs "Separates" list continued at the back

Leadership and Organization for Community Prevention and Intervention in Venezuela

Maritza Montero, PhD
Editor

Leadership and Organization for Community Prevention and Intervention in Venezuela has been co-published simultaneously as *Journal of Prevention & Intervention in the Community*, Volume 27, Number 1 2004.

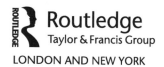

Routledge
Taylor & Francis Group

LONDON AND NEW YORK

First published 2004 by The Haworth Press, Inc.

2 Park Square, Milton Park, Abingdon, Oxfordshire OX14 4RN
605 Third Avenue, New York, NY 10017

Routledge is an imprint of the Taylor & Francis Group, an informa business

First issued in paperback 2020

Copyright © 2004 Taylor & Francis

Leadership and Organization for Community Prevention and Intervention in Venezuela has been co-published simultaneously as *Journal of Prevention & Intervention in the Community*™, Volume 27, Number 1 2004.

Cover design by Jennifer Gaska

Library of Congress Cataloging-in-Publication Data

Leadership and organization for community prevention and intervention in Venezuela / Maritza Montero, editor.
     p. cm.
     "Co-published simultaneously as Journal of prevention & intervention in the community, volume 27, number 1."
     Includes bibliographical references and index.
     ISBN 0-7890-1248-0 (hard cover : alk. paper) – ISBN 0-7890-1513-7 (soft cover : alk. paper)
     1. Community leadership–Venezuela. 2. Community organization–Venezuela. 3. Community development–Venezuela. I. Montero, Maritza. II. Journal of prevention & intervention in the community.
HN370.Z9C65 2003
307–dc22

                                                2003022961

ISBN 978-0-7890-1513-6 (pbk)

Indexing, Abstracting & Website/Internet Coverage

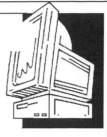

This section provides you with a list of major indexing & abstracting services. That is to say, each service began covering this periodical during the year noted in the right column. Most Websites which are listed below have indicated that they will either post, disseminate, compile, archive, cite or alert their own Website users with research-based content from this work. (This list is as current as the copyright date of this publication.)

Abstracting, Website/Indexing Coverage . . . . Year When Coverage Began

- *Behavioral Medicine Abstracts* **1996**

- *CAB Abstracts c/o CAB International/CAB ACCESS. . . available in print, disketts updated weekly, and on Internet. Providing full bibliographic listings, author affiliation, augmented keyword searching <http://www.cabi.org/>* **2004**

- *CINAHL (Cumulative Index to Nursing & Allied Health Literature), in print, EBSCO, and Silverplatter, Data-Star, and PaperChase. (Support materials include Subject Heading List, Database Search Guide, and instructional video). <http://www.cinahl.com>* **2003**

- *CNPIEC Reference Guide: Chinese National Directory of Foreign Periodicals* **1996**

- *Educational Research Abstracts (ERA) (online database) <http://www.tandf.co.uk/era>* **2002**

- *EMBASE/Excerpta Medica Secondary Publishing Division <http://www.elsevier.nl>* **1996**

- *e-psyche, LLC <http://www.e-psyche.net>* **2001**

- *Family Index Database <http://www.familyscholar.com>* **2003**

(continued)

(continued)

*Special Bibliographic Notes related to special journal issues
(separates) and indexing/abstracting:*

- indexing/abstracting services in this list will also cover material in any "separate" that is co-published simultaneously with Haworth's special thematic journal issue or DocuSerial. Indexing/abstracting usually covers material at the article/chapter level.
- monographic co-editions are intended for either non-subscribers or libraries which intend to purchase a second copy for their circulating collections.
- monographic co-editions are reported to all jobbers/wholesalers/approval plans. The source journal is listed as the "series" to assist the prevention of duplicate purchasing in the same manner utilized for books-in-series.
- to facilitate user/access services all indexing/abstracting services are encouraged to utilize the co-indexing entry note indicated at the bottom of the first page of each article/chapter/contribution.
- this is intended to assist a library user of any reference tool (whether print, electronic, online, or CD-ROM) to locate the monographic version if the library has purchased this version but not a subscription to the source journal.
- individual articles/chapters in any Haworth publication are also available through the Haworth Document Delivery Service (HDDS).

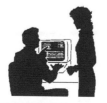

Leadership and Organization for Community Prevention and Intervention in Venezuela

CONTENTS

ABOUT THE EDITOR

Maritza Montero, PhD, is Professor and Coordinator of Psychology Doctorate Studies at Universidad Central de Venezuela. She received her MSc in Psychology from Universidad "Simon Bolivar," in Venezuela and her PhD in Sociology from Universite de Paris in France. Dr. Montero is the co-founder of the Venezuelan Social Psychology Association and founder of "Constelacion Venezolana," a community program that incorporates art and reflection and is designed to empower children from low-income and urban poverty zones. She has published several books and papers on community psychology and is an associate editor of the *American Journal of Community Psychology* and a member of the editorial boards of the *Journal of Community Psychology* and *Community Work and Family,* among others. In 2000 Dr. Montero received the Venezuelan National Social Science Award, and in 1995 she received the Interamerican Society of Psychology Award.

Community Organization
and Leadership in Venezuela:
A Prologue

Irma Serrano-García

University of Puerto Rico

What does one look for when one reads an article, a special issue, a book? Usually one is seeking new ideas, answers to questions and new challenges. I have always found that the text is particularly exciting if it poses more questions than it answers because in that manner it creates the path for new quests, for reflections on usual practices, for new beginnings. This volume edited by Maritza Montero meets these standards. I will try to briefly examine its contributions to the theme of community organization and leadership and particularly to identify the questions it raised for me so as to provoke the reader to seek new answers.

Various authors refer to the concept of community. They stress the notion that this concept has evolved from being limited by locality and geographical boundaries to being defined by relationships, functionality and sense of belonging. They mention how this is even more palpable at present when the frontiers of our communities are expanded by the impact of globalization and technology. Although for some time now this issue has been raised (Chavis & Newbrough, 1986; Durham, 1986; Krause, 2001), it is particularly important to re-examine it in a format whose focus is community prevention and research. What does this expanded definition mean for community efforts? What impact does it have on how we examine leadership and organization?

[Haworth co-indexing entry note]: "Community Organization and Leadership in Venezuela: A Prologue." Serrano-García, Irma. Co-published simultaneously in *Journal of Prevention & Intervention in the Community* (The Haworth Press, Inc.) Vol. 27, No. 1, 2004, pp. xv-xix; and: *Leadership and Organization for Community Prevention and Intervention in Venezuela* (ed: Maritza Montero) The Haworth Press, Inc., 2004, pp. xiii-xvii. Single or multiple copies of this article are available for a fee from The Haworth Document Delivery Service [1-800-HAWORTH, 9:00 a.m. - 5:00 p.m. (EST). E-mail address: docdelivery@haworthpress.com].

On the other hand, all chapters in the book focus on geographical communities–Casalta; Urban working class communities; Low-income communities in Caracas; Las Minitas, Raúl Leoni II, Blandín, Las Torres. Is the expanded definition of community evident in these efforts? Have the concepts of leadership and organization changed as we change our conceptualization of community?

The concept of leadership is examined thoroughly. Various important contributions are forwarded. Sánchez, Montero and Lodo-Platone stress the importance of participation as a correlate of leadership, dwell on the inseparability of leaders and others (they prefer not to call them followers) and stress how participatory leadership is the purview of community settings, versus formal or traditional organizations. They present contrasting characteristics or features of leaders in these settings. Montero, in a provocative and down-to-earth way, also presents a typology of community leadership which is quite distinct from the usual categories we are used to seeing in the literature (i.e., democratic, authoritative, laissez-faire; Cartwright & Zander, 1980). The thrust of these articles is that communities, and in particular communities with a participatory "tradition," generate or require different kinds of leaders. Leaders in other settings are bound by structure and established norms.

Although the analysis is sound and convincing within the exposed contexts, I wonder if the participatory and altruistic leaders they describe can only arise in these settings. Can we not create formal organizations which allow for this kind of leadership? If the creation of settings is a strategy favored by common psychologists (Sarason, 1972, 1997; Cherniss & Deegan, 2000), can we not incorporate these reflections into the development of alternative scenarios?

All authors are not, however, unified behind this participatory leadership concept. There are some contradictions in this volume , as should be. Farías and Perdomo make a significant contribution on examining the ethical and moral dilemmas that community leaders face, although further description of each dilemma would have been desirable. This is much-needed work since most of the writing regarding ethics and morals impose on community workers the definitions and solutions of ethical/moral conflicts developed for individual level interventions (Snow, Grady, & Goyette-Ewing, 2000). Hernández adds important ideas regarding leadership development and training and the importance of self-reflection in the process. This is compatible with both Montero's and Sánchez's argument that the participatory leader facilitates constant reflection in his/her settings. However, both Farías and Perdomo and Hernández seem to focus on a more traditional definition of leader, one who is more distant from others than Sánchez and Montero would wish. This is exemplified by training sessions exclusively for leaders (without their followers) and by the moral dilemma of a choice between being paternalistic or facilitating empowerment. If we wanted to foster the development of participatory leadership in community settings, should Hernández's training sessions change? What new moral or ethical issues do participatory leaders have to face?

Lodo-Platone's contribution is unique since it examines how other community structures, in this case the family, impact community life and would have to be taken into account by any responsible, committed community leader. She also presents the relationship of the community to government services and the mediators between them. She illustrates how it is essential to understand community dynamics and characteristics so as to develop community organization efforts.

The authors in this volume make other contributions that are not directly specified as related to the subject matter. Interdisciplinary contributions are evident in their work. Sánchez uses organizational theory, Montero refers to the social psychological literature on leadership, Farías and Perdomo present developmental psychology concepts, Lodo-Platone refers to the literature on family functioning and Hernández focuses on cognitive and behavioral models. Not since Rappaport's (1977) seminal chapter on "Conceptions for Individual Psychology Useful to the Community Psychologist" have I seen so evident an integration of other disciplinary contributions to that of community work.

Within this same thread of thought, the focus on emotions seemed particularly significant. Various authors refer to the emotional component of leadership, to the emotions that emerge, facilitate or hinder community efforts. In a scientific world where most contributions separate our feelings from our ideas (Varas-Diáz & Serrano-García, 2003), this emphasis is refreshing and more true-to-life. It also allows us to consider questions such as: How can we harness our emotions so they become our allies in community work? How can recognizing the emotional side of organizing facilitate participatory leadership and the creation of more flexible and accessible human service settings?

Another issue which is touched upon in various papers merits attention. Montero states that most community leaders are women and Lodo-Platone indicates the centrality of women in family and community dynamics. Although some could argue that this phenomenon is context-specific, in other words that this occurs only in Venezuela, my experience is that this happens in most Latin American countries and in many minority communities in the U.S. Considering what we know of gender relations and power structures (Jenkins, 2000; Sagestrano, 1992), what does this imply for community efforts? Does the feminization of community work have a direct impact on the development of participatory models of leadership? Does it have a favorable or deleterious impact on their capacity to mobilize others? On their capacity to confront the powers that be? On the kind of organizational structures that arise? I find these questions a fascinating area for further research and action.

A similar issue arises when various authors refer to the religiousness of participatory or altruistic leaders, or to the importance of religion (organized or not) on community life. Is this also a local or context-bound issue? Does this also influence the nature of leadership organization and effectiveness of community work? Various authors in the U.S. have started to work on this issue (Maton & Pargament, 1987; Pargament & Maton, 2000). I do not know of concerted efforts to examine it in Latin American countries.

Various authors also refer to the hardships of community leadership. Montero and Sánchez mention how it is hard to motivate people to accept this role and of the personal sacrifices it requires which makes it difficult to maintain for long periods of time. Lodo-Platone mentions the fragility of community involvement. Are these hardships more or less for participatory leaders? Is generating, facilitating and maintaining participation more of a task than those which traditional leaders have to face? Does it, however, generate enough support to sustain involvement and commitment? These are all empirical questions.

Finally, a note on research methods. All articles in this volume use qualitative research masterfully. Some use ethnographic methods, others use qualitative interviews, diaries, and field notes. I believe, as I know do the authors, that this gives one a deeper understanding of communal, organizational and individual realities. However, is there no space for quantitative methods in this subject of research? For mixed-methods? What kinds of questions could be asked and answered with these strategies that qualitative methods do not respond to?

In summary, I believe this is a thought-provoking piece. It has contributed to my ideas and feelings about community, leadership, organization, interdisciplinary work, and research. It has raised many questions and helped me identify new areas of interest. I challenge you all to read it carefully and chart a steady course toward the exploration of these new or partially explored worlds.

REFERENCES

Cartwright, D. & Zander, A. (1980). *Dinámica de grupos: Investigación y teoría.* México, D.F., México: Trillas.

Chavis, D. M. & Newbrough, J. R. (1986). The meaning of "community" in community psychology. *Journal of Community Psychology, 14,* 335-340.

Cherniss, C. & Deegan, G. (2000). The creation of alternative settings. In J. Rappaport & E. Seidman (2000) (Eds.). *Handbook of Community Psychology.* (359-377). New York, NY: Kluwer/Academic/Plenum Pub.

Durham, H. W. (1986). Commentary. The community today: Place or process. *Journal of Community Psychology, 14,* 399-404.

Jenkins, S. (2000). Introduction to the special issue: Defining gender, relationships and power. *Sex Roles, 42* (7/8), 467-493.

Krause, M. (2001). Hacia una redefinición del concepto de comunidad; Cuatro ejes para un análisis crítico y una propuesta. *Revista de Psicologaía, X*(2), 49 60.

Maton, K. & Pargament, K. (1987) The roles of religion in prevention and promotion. *Prevention in Human Services, 3,* 37-72.

Pargament, K. & Maton, K. (2000) Religion in American life. In J. Rappaport & E. Seidman (2000) (Eds.). *Handbook of Community Psychology.* (495-522). New York, NY: Kluwer/Academic/Plenum Pub.

Rappaport, J. (1977). *Community psychology: Values, action and research.* New York, NY: Holt, Rinehart & Winston.

Sagestrano, L. (1992). The use of power and influence in a gendered world. *Psychology of Women Quarterly, 16,* 439-447.

Sarason, S. (1972). *The creation of settings and the future societies.* San Francisco, CA: Jossey-Bass.

Sarason, S. (1997). Revisiting the creation of settings. *Mind, culture and activity, 4* (3),175-182.

Snow, D., Grady, K., & Goyette-Ewing, M. (2000). A perspective on ethical issues in community psychology. In J. Rappaport & E. Seidman (2000) (Eds.). *Handbook of Community Psychology.* (897-917). New York, NY: Kluwer/Academic/Plenum Pub.

Varas-Díaz, N. & Serrano-García, I. (2002). ¿Pensabas que emocionarse era sencillo?: Las emociones como fenómenos biológicos, cognoscitivos y sociales. *Revista Puertorriqueña de Psicologia, 13,* 9-28.

Presentation

Maritza Montero

Universidad Central de Venezuela

Theories of leadership speak about certain types of leaders: authoritarian, democratic, laissez-faire; there are trait, situational and contingency explanations for leadership, but psychosocial community work provides experiences that need to be examined from the community's own perspective. As can be seen in the papers in this volume, the categories attributed to several of those categories of leadership can be found coinciding in the same leader, and interesting forms of relation between leaders and not exactly "followers," but co-participants, are observed everyday in community research and action. Every community has leaders. They, along with most of the people in those communities, give it some form of organisation.

This does not mean that those leaders are to be considered as special figures necessarily placed above their fellow community members, even when sometimes that may happen. Community leaders can spontaneously arise according to the activities that need to be carried out, according to the occasion; and it is not a matter of age, or gender or social status, but of capacity, commitment, and the group's acceptation. They appear and disappear in many community-managed development programmes. And as will be seen in the papers composing this volume, the kind of leadership being presented is characterised by its predominantly participatory condition.

[Haworth co-indexing entry note]: "Presentation." Montero, Maritza. Co-published simultaneously in *Journal of Prevention & Intervention in the Community* (The Haworth Press, Inc.) Vol. 27, No. 1, 2004, pp. 1-5; and: *Leadership and Organization for Community Prevention and Intervention in Venezuela* (ed: Maritza Montero) The Haworth Press, Inc., 2004, pp. 1-5. Single or multiple copies of this article are available for a fee from The Haworth Document Delivery Service [1-800-HAWORTH, 9:00 a.m. - 5:00 p.m. (EST). E-mail address: docdelivery@haworthpress.com].

Venezuela, the country where the five studies in this volume were carried out, has a tradition of community work going back to the late sixties, although the community psychosocial perspective was introduced in the late seventies.

At the beginning, the main sources were governmental social programmes, followed later by the studies simultaneously coming from academic institutions and NGOs with missions directed towards social development. Although the governmental programmes of the late 60s and the 70s were markedly populist in character, and were plagued by political clientelism; at the same time, they were large well-financed projects. Actually, two institutions were created to conduct the Venezuelan government community social policies: Fundacomún and Fundasocial, both foundations directed to develop and support community organisations and social programmes concerning them, based on the idea that social development should incorporate the people.

Along with their political partisan intention they also produced a positive effect: the population became aware that the people united in community participation can achieve certain effects favourable to all. Organisation, participation and leadership became accessible to ordinary people, who came to see them as activities within their reach. And at the same time, those activities received legal regulation within special laws recognising and protecting certain community organisations such as the neighbours' associations. So, if on one hand the policy implementation was used to favour the political party with the reins of the government, community action also became an alternative mode of political action and a new political arena, because as a space was created for citizen participation, and it became accosted and invaded by political parties, the citizens integrating the communities had the experience of doing things together, and producing changes. Today we can see in some low-income sectors (*barrios*) of Venezuelan main cities, streets or alleys with the names of those pioneers of community organisation that led movements directed to build roads, or bring services to those places.

A community culture is being constructed incorporating into Venezuelan quotidian life the idea of the possibilities residing in the joint efforts carried out by people united not only by the sharing of a certain space, but also, and very importantly, by the sharing of a life lived in common, where certain circumstances have affected a group of persons producing at the same time different reactions, and the same benefits or problems. Although most of the psychosocial community work being done in the country has had as target low-income or marginalised communities, one can find very effective community organisations in the higher income communities, which have managed to privatise some streets and roads, closing them to free public transit, in the name of security. That culture then has served as a partisan banner, and as a way to introduce desired changes within communities (i.e., environmental, organizational, in the quality of life), reflecting their social expectations.

A corpus of systematic information shows some tendencies concerning community leadership and organisation, among which are the following:

1. Most community leaders are women and this is so in both urban and rural areas.
2. Age of community leaders covers an ample range: middle-aged and old people do not predominate. Frequently, some of the leaders have evolved from directing child and teen-age groups (sports, play) to leading community organisations.
3. Even though community leadership is a phenomenon in which traditional classifications can be reflected, it surpasses them and presents elements pertaining to the circumstances where it originates.
4. Authoritarian or domineering forms of leadership are accompanied by important affective elements. Rejection of authoritarian forms of leadership is an example: passivity and withdrawal from community programmes go together with affective manifestations and some sort of subdued critique and disqualifying mockery.
5. Community leadership positions have not as many people desiring to occupy them as could be expected. In fact, the level of commitment and work that comes with them is the cause of avoidance in some communities.

Euclides Sánchez's paper presents a view of how that community culture is expressed. The people at the Casalta Project, who managed to build six housing units (buildings) going from a refuge for the homeless (they had lost their shanties in the hills, taken away by mudslides), to organised action leading to comfortable flats, debated, discussed, thought and worked. From his experience with that project, Sánchez presents several propositions showing how the interaction in a participatory organised community produces and is produced by an inclusive, flexible, reflective leadership, visible, accessible, committed, effective and also dispensable. The singularity of the phenomenon described, illustrated by the opinions of the participants, resides in the participatory character of the experience.

Farías and Perdomo address leadership from the perspective of the leaders, specifically those characterised by their altruism, and the moral dilemmas they confront. These authors relate the leaders' moral development and their sense of community, discussing the limits and scope of individual and community perspectives regarding this topic. The four persons that worked with Farías and Perdomo are no ordinary leaders; their behaviour and reasoning about their relation to the community and the people integrating it seems to provide a view of morality wider than the models usually studying it.

Eneiza Hernández describes an intervention carried out with community leaders directed to provide them with some tools to make their decisions within the community more efficient and more adequate to the task and circumstances they have to address. She introduces the concept of metadecision (thinking and reflecting about their decision-making), presenting how reflective and critical training workshops increased their awareness about the cognitive and interactive tools available, and how to use them, becoming more conscious about the meaning of their decisions and the affective aspects involved.

Maria Luisa Lodo-Platone presents an ethnographic and psychosocial description of the role played and interaction maintained by families within the community, and how they contribute to, and at the same time support and are supported by, community organisation. The network of interrelations they create facilitates daily life, creating a sort of intermediate level of organisation facilitating daily life in the barrio communities.

Finally, my own work deals with different modes of exerting community leadership encountered during my psychosocial community research and action: altruistic leaders such as those interviewed by Farías and Perdomo (I have worked with the two women leaders he interviewed); trasformational leaders such as those discussed by the Casalta people in the Sánchez paper; and also, the difficult narcissistic leaders that can be exasperating and worrisome, but also, sometimes charming, that belong to the communities we work with, and as part of them it is inevitable to deal with them.

Each community is unique, some communities have things in common, and at the analytical level, the concepts tend to unify the community perspectives we study into those systematic explanatory constructions called theories. Observing what happens in the communities and reflecting about that with their members, studying them, we can produce some knowledge that perhaps can be useful for other communities, and for their internal and external agents. These five Venezuelan experiences present a view of community leadership and organisation that has provided their authors wide grounds for reflection. We have learned while doing these researches, and we want to share with another community what we have learned. This new community is that of the psychologists in a wider world. If a dialogue is produced, we shall be very happy to further increase our learning from the exchange.

Maritza Montero
Caracas, Venezuela
March 2003

Organization and Leadership in the Participatory Community

Euclides Sánchez

Universidad Central de Venezuela

SUMMARY. Participation is a community mobilization process which develops in relation to its internal and external conditions. Two of the most salient internal conditions due to their importance for the development of community participation (CP) are the organization and the leadership adopted by participants throughout the participatory project. That is, the community constructs along its self-management process, the particularities that those conditions should have, so that they correspond with the meaning of participation orienting it and with the characteristics of the goals the community attempts to achieve. It is argued that organization and leadership develop in the participatory community not only as related conditions, as they jointly influence CP, but as two conditions which mutually influence one another, so that the definition the community makes of one of them converges with the definition of the other one. That relationship is examined taking as illustration a case study of CP which has a successful history of seventeen years of continued participation. *[Article copies available for a fee from The Haworth Document Delivery Service: 1-800-HAWORTH. E-mail address: <docdelivery@haworthpress.com> Website: <http://www.HaworthPress.com> © 2004 by The Haworth Press, Inc. All rights reserved.]*

Euclides Sánchez is affiliated with the Universidad Central de Venezuela, Instituto de Psicología, Apdo. 47018, Caracas, 1041-A, Venezuela (E-mail: eusanche@reacciun.ve).

[Haworth co-indexing entry note]: "Organization and Leadership in the Participatory Community." Sánchez, Euclides. Co-published simultaneously in *Journal of Prevention & Intervention in the Community* (The Haworth Press, Inc.) Vol. 27, No. 1, 2004, pp. 7-23; and: *Leadership and Organization for Community Prevention and Intervention in Venezuela* (ed: Maritza Montero) The Haworth Press, Inc., 2004, pp. 7-23. Single or multiple copies of this article are available for a fee from The Haworth Document Delivery Service [1-800-HAWORTH, 9:00 a.m. - 5:00 p.m. (EST). E-mail address: docdelivery@haworthpress.com].

KEYWORDS. Participation, community, organization, leadership

The title *Organization and Leadership in the Participatory Community* (PC) assumes that the characteristics of organization and leadership in communities of this kind differ from those found in other social organizations. This work reflects that assumption; it seeks to show the particular characteristics that these two processes acquire in PCs, through reliance on analysis of the information generated by a case of community participation (CP) in which there is already a history of over 20 years of successful participation in addressing community issues.

The term organization is understood as the way in which the community's activities are co-ordinated in the different stages of development of its participatory experience, with the aim of achieving the goals adopted by the group. Leadership is conceived as the process of direction through which the community's actions were guided. Having defined those two concepts, and before proceeding to describe the case, it is necessary to indicate what we mean by community and participation, so as to enhance understanding of the conceptual framework in which we place PC.

DEFINITION OF COMMUNITY

According to Hunter and Riger (1986), one criterion on which the definition of community has been based is geographic in nature: the characterization of community interaction in terms of its spatial location. Agreement on this score is reflected in such old definitions of community as: "In a broad sense, the concept of community is used to designate social units with certain social characteristics that endow it with an organization within a given *area*" [italics added] (Pozas, 1964, p. 21), or "the approach that tends to prevail is the one that considers the community as a group whose components occupy a *territory* [italics added] within which the entire life cycle can play out" (Chinoy, 1968, p. 61), or more recently, "a community is a dynamic, historical, and culturally constituted and developed social group, whose existence precedes the arrival of the researchers or social interveners, in which interests, objectives, needs, and problems are shared, in a given *space* [italics added] and time, which collectively generates an identity, along with organizational forms, and developing and using resources for its ends" (Montero, 1998, p. 2).

However, Hunter and Riger (1986) assert that community is not just the result of a reference to a place, but also that of interests which do not necessarily have a spatial location; the logical implication is that a person can belong to several communities at once. Heller (1989) takes a similar position, stating that a community should not be understood solely as a locality. For this author, the spatial identifier was initially useful to facilitate commercial relations among the sources of products, transportation, and users, but with the growth of cities, communities have become increasingly complex and citizens have also come to associate on the basis of other issues that unite them. Heller prefers to speak of "community as a relation" in order to highlight the quality of human interaction, the social bonds that develop among individuals. What counts is the community as interaction, as social cohesion.

In spite of the foregoing critiques of the spatial dimension for identifying community, this criterion still helps to designate groups of inhabitants who are linked to specific surroundings–even though the growth of cities has undoubtedly weakened those links. This position coincides with that of Moreno (1996), who says in reference to lower-income urban communities: "Living together in a given neighborhood, which implies a certain *territory* [italics added], may have been the minimum feature common to all our communities; accordingly, the neighborhood or a specific segment of it is the typical community in a city . . ." (p. 49). And Durham (1986) admits that though community has changed from a place to a process, the place dimension continues to exist, even if it exerts less influence than in the past.

Based on these arguments, we might conclude that the concept of community is a broader one, and its definition should focus on some kind of unifying element that embraces the community as both a locality and a relationship. This is just what Chavis and Newbrough (1986) intend when they define community as "the set of social relations that are interlinked by a feeling of community" (p. 335).

According to this approach, then, what distinguishes a community from any other social grouping–whether it has a specific territory or not–is the overall feeling of belonging, of solidarity and trust in the value of the collective dimension that is implicit in the expression *community feeling*, defined by McMillan and Chavis (1986) as: "a feeling that the members have about their membership, a feeling that the members are concerned about each other and the group is concerned about them, and a shared faith that their needs will be met by staying together" (p. 9).

In other words, according to these formulations, community is based on the components of membership or a feeling of sharing personal relations with others, an individual's influence or possibility of exerting influence over the group or vice versa, a common perception of needs that are jointly addressed in order to meet them, and a shared emotional bond through which the members feel the group, the place, the time, and their experience to be common to all.

Community and the community feeling are not, however, separate concepts–even though that is the impression that emerges from a review of the literature. Rather, community feeling is a part of the definition of community (Hubert, 1996). Put another way, a community is a social organization that is determined by the quality of its membership, the reciprocal influence between the group and its members, who share and work together to solve their problems, and whose members feel affectively related; these are the components of the feeling of community.

AN IDEA OF COMMUNITY PARTICIPATION

We prefer to speak of the idea of CP rather than a definition of it, since CP is today a type of community mobilization which changes so rapidly that any definition of it runs the risk of quickly being rendered incomplete. The expression *idea of*, on the contrary, is transitory in nature, and open to the incorporation of new elements. In this respect, and following Sánchez (2000), we view PC as a process of voluntary and inclusive collective action whereby a community engages in an organized pursuit of common goals; that generally implies exerting an influence on government decisions which affect the scope of those goals in one way or another.

When we say CP is a process we mean that it is not a steady state but a process that creates itself over time, during which the participants acquire and train others in the use of particular knowledge and skills that vary with the nature of their participatory experience. The assertion that participation is not a stable entity also implies a recognition of its variability according to the elements which make up the context and the time in which that experience takes place. In other words, the process of participation is built up on the basis of the interaction among the characteristics of the participating group (such as its experience in participation, its level and form of organization, its leadership, the resources at its disposal to strive for a solution of the problem that motivates it), the nature of the project on which it has embarked (for example, a role in the formulation of a social security policy, self-help housing construction, renovation of a lower-income neighborhood, or lobbying for public health or educational services), access to and control over the resources needed, and the political climate towards participation.

In this kind of relationship it is the participants themselves who, in an ongoing interaction among themselves and with the other components of the process, build up what their participation consists of, over time. The meaning of participation as it develops, congruently with the actions taken, is therefore influenced by the quality of the participatory experience and it will therefore differ from one such experience to the next. Participation is not, then, "something" of a universal nature; it is rather a social construction of multiple dimensions, subject to the values and contextual circumstances prevailing at a given time.

CP, on the other hand, has ends which orient it: the achievement of goals on which the group reaches agreement reflecting their importance to the satisfaction of vital interests–by which we mean interests so important as to mobilize the group members to perform actions requiring perseverance over time and diversity of content.

In addition, given the tension between the citizens' needs and values and the State's control over the resources required for their satisfaction, as well as the State's tendency to apply its own scheme of values in addressing those needs, the community aspires through its participation to play a role in public decision making which affects it. For that reason, and due to the collective nature of the objectives the community pursues, participation cannot be an individual process; it must be an organized collective process.

Finally, participation is a voluntary act which expresses the development of awareness of the value of participatory action, and hence, of the need for solidarity among peers. But at the same time, it wishes that awareness to spread to all the members of the community, with the result that more and more members come to participate. This quality imbues participation with an inclusive dimension, thereby ensuring minority groups' right to make themselves heard in the participatory project.

CP, in a nutshell, is a process that leads to intercession in the public decision-making process, even if that is not the goal around which the community initially mobilizes. It could be said that the original motive for community action is the solution of a concrete problem, i.e., a search for a material benefit. But it is through reflection on participatory action that CP stimulates the community to redefine its original needs and the ways to seek their satisfaction. These new constructions that are influenced by the specificity of the community's values are not congruent with the general conception with which the State imbues its policies and programs. Hence, in its relations with the decision-making organs the community–through its participation–creates an opportunity for its alternative view to be carried into reality. The following citation is an eloquent expression of this process:

> Look, the thing is that participation is not just asking for benefits . . . ,
> that's how it begins . . . , what do you think, that a person . . . that
> people, don't think? Look, people speak, debate, hold meetings,
> talk at home, and even the kids give their opinions, . . . , people discuss everything: the insecurity problem, celebration of Mother's
> Day. . . . Look, do you think that if we had not debated, thought,
> and fought for what is ours, we would have Casalta? No. We
> would surely be living in a barracks as displaced people, which is
> what the government offered us . . . temporarily they said. That is
> asking for benefits, but the other thing, reflection, also comes
> along, that is participation.[1]

THE CASE STUDY

The community studied, called *La Esperanza* or *The Casalta Project*, got its start in September 1980 when a group of 39 lower-income families living in the west side of Caracas lost their homes to a landslide on the hill where they had lived. Thereafter the families organized and commenced a CP process through which they obtained economic assistance from the local government and advising from the Central University of Venezuela to carry out a self-help housing construction project. The project culminated in the construction of 69 apartments, in which an equal number of families now live.

But community participation did not stop with the completion of housing construction; it has continued to this day. This feature makes Casalta an interesting case of continuity of CP, since it is common for communities to interrupt their participatory experiences.

The information on the characteristics of the community's organization and leadership was collected mainly through semi-structured interviews with 13 participants of both sexes. The qualitative analysis of the data was performed using the ATLAS-ti computer program.[2]

ORGANIZATION AND LEADERSHIP IN THE COMMUNITY

The results generated by that analysis point to a set of characteristics of community organization and leadership in *La Esperanza*, which are described here in the form of propositional statements.

Regarding Organization

First Proposition

The PC's organization was not imposed, but emerged from the pattern of participation adopted by the community. CP oscillates over the course of its development, its variation being influenced by the changes in the community's internal conditions, the nature of the goals it has addressed, and the competence of its leaders, or by external conditions such as the support of government agencies. But as its CP changes, the PC modifies its organizational structure to adapt it to new requirements for participation.

Two examples drawn from the case in point illustrate this proposition. The first refers to the project's beginnings, during which the design of the new housing units, the type of support forthcoming from the State, and the advising that would be given by the Central University of Venezuela had to be decided upon. As was to be expected, community participation in this period was largely focused on an assessment of the different options offered by the city government to overcome the lack of housing; this required the community to keep itself informed about those options at all times. To meet this demand, the community agreed to include a weekly general meeting in its organizational structure. That meeting became the stage on which the community leaders informed the members on the project's progress and in which the members had a chance to take part in the decisions that were being made. This macro level of organization had to be complemented with a micro level, comprised of working groups that carried out the decisions made at the general meetings.

The second example comes from the community's present-day life. Community participation at the present time focuses mainly on maintenance of the housing units and activities intended to strengthen families and enhance the members' cultural level. Hence, the community organization has been restructured as follows: a condominium board for each building that oversees its maintenance, and a governing council comprising two delegates from each building and the community board of directors, which meets at weekly intervals. The council meetings are open, allowing the other community members to attend and make statements and proposals in what is termed the "miscellaneous" part of the agenda.

Another current community goal is to see that CP is continued by the successor generations through the creation of opportunities for young people to take part in decision making. The new organizational structure allots three seats on the Board of Directors to youths from the community.

Second Proposition

The PC's organization acknowledges CP's inclusive nature. As stated in our discussion of the idea of participation, CP implies an acknowledgment of involvement by all sectors of the community, regardless of the specific characteristics that distinguish them. In this regard, and reflecting the participatory project's requirements, the PC's organization must provide mechanisms to facilitate the participation of both sexes and different age groups, including the community members whose time is limited or those subject to any other restrictions. The working groups organized in Casalta had mixed membership, even for construction work, and flexible time schedules for self-help housing construction. As a result, all the families could put in the 40 hours per week that the community had determined as the minimum family obligation.

Third Proposition

The PC's organization is a flexible one, which seeks to satisfy the community members' specific and general reasons for participating. CP is a process that mobilizes new visions and new interests among the participants. For example, they often express interest in changing their participatory activity or in simultaneously participating in a number of different tasks.

It was found in Casalta that, as the project advanced, the community members felt increasingly attracted to the acquisition of skills as varied as learning how to speak at meetings or learning welding techniques. The community's organizational mechanisms permitted the satisfaction of that variety of interests, since the members could rotate among working groups or participate in several of them at the same time.

Fourth Proposition

The PC's organization facilitates reflection on participation itself. CP is a learning process in which the participant transforms him or herself while transforming his or her environment. But this implies that the community members must have opportunities for reflection, in which they critically examine their actions and assess the different components of the participatory process (such as its organization, leadership, goals, and member involvement). This reflection stimulates the participants to elaborate new meanings regarding their roles in the participatory project, proactive strategies to achieve the stated goals, and the responsibility of the other agents involved in the project's success or failure. The outcome of this process is what Kieffer (1984) terms the cycle of practice, or "the circular relationship between experience and reflection" (p. 26).

In Casalta, the key opportunity for reflection in the project's first stage was the general meeting, where all the community members could freely debate the project's progress. In the current stage, the Governing Council and the periodic community general meetings provide that opportunity for reflection.

Regarding Leadership

First Proposition

The PC's leaders are visible and accessible. They are leaders who are easy for the community members to find and approach. They do not pose obstacles to access when someone wants to express an idea that might improve the project's progress or discuss problems that inhibit it. Following are examples of this openness:

Q. How did you, or anyone coming into the community, know who the leaders were?

A. That was no problem. They were not only the people we elected, but also, they never hid. They were always there, at the general meeting, working with the people.[1]

Q. How could you approach the leaders, to communicate something or to express a difference of opinion vs. theirs?

A. Easy, because they were always there, they were always available, always concerned with you, at their battle stations. They never tried to distance themselves, even when someone went to criticize them.[1]

Second Proposition

They have multiple areas of competence:

1. In courage:

   [Our leaders] were the most knowledgeable, the boldest, well, you sat down at their feet: "Are we going to move?" "We're going to move!" Sometimes they made you feel afraid, or nervous, but when they showed the courage they had, you followed them, you felt yourself filled up with energy.[1]

2. In experience with community work:

   [W]hen the time came to speak, they were the ones who had the most experience in going to the government, to lead the community.[1]

3. In generating good ideas for the community:

   The people in the community contributed good ideas for the project, but the leaders were out front. Their ideas were always good.[1]

4. In stimulating participation by the community members:

   [The leaders] stimulated the people to participate, because many people had stage fright and didn't want to say what they felt, so it was easier to ask what everyone felt about any situation. More concretely, about the State's proposals.[1]

5. In the use of effective strategies for communication with the community:

   We were bread and coffee, [though] we were people displaced by a disaster. There they were [the leaders], they spoke. They didn't just say: "We're going to do this and that." No, they called on the people, they talked to them, they explained things, they explained things to you: "All right, what do you think? Are we going to do it? Do you agree? Do you disagree?" The most natural thing in the world, and generally for everyone, with everyone participating in what they were doing, in what they were achieving.[1]

Third Proposition

The PC's leadership shares with the other community members. The PC builds the concept of leadership as a shared condition, i.e., as a condition common to all participants without distinction.

> [T]he leaders weren't the ones who really directed the entire community, because the Board looked for a person responsible for the bathroom, . . . a person responsible for the day and night shifts, and the general meeting was the one to make the decisions. So it was the community that directed.[1]

Fourth Proposition

The PC's leaders are necessary and dispensable at the same time. The PC acknowledges the importance of having leaders who accept the responsibility of orienting the group's activity. However, precisely due to the shared nature of leadership, the community does not fall into a dependence on particular leaders, but has the ability to replace them with new leaders when circumstances warrant.

> If . . . these people hadn't been there, well, we were a fuse that was out and we needed a match to light us.[1]

> The thing is that if the fighters for the community as a whole had been others, things would have gone just as well because we were all organized, that is, the members of the Board of Directors were appointed by the community, and well, if they had been other people, as long as they came from the community, everything would have been just the same.[1]

To sum up, the PC's organization is what could be described as a democratic organization because it respects and complies with the membership's decisions, and a participatory one because it is the outcome thereof. As one member of the Casalta community put it:

> A lot of people who don't vote in national elections vote here, because they feel this is their organization, their government.

On the other hand, the PC's organization is a meaning that is constructed. It is a structure of functions built up by the community in accordance with its needs and values. It is, therefore, an organization legitimated by and in participation; that is what endows it with a participatory-democratic character.

If we contrast this assertion with what happens in capital-producing organizations or formal organizations, we would probably find that they do not have that character, but, rather, are marked by the acceptance of a pre-existing organizational structure. We may wonder, however, whether that is valid for all their components. In any event, and bearing in mind the differences between the two classes of organizations, as in collective definition of goals, at this point we might well question the adequacy of the existing conceptualizations of organizational functioning–largely drawn from the study of formal organizations–to yield an understanding of organizations called voluntary.

Leadership in a PC is a leadership that is grounded in the foundations of visibility, accessibility, and competence in communicating with the community and fostering its members' participation. In the second place, it is a leadership that shares the decision-making function. This attribute of shared leadership, which could be termed participatory leadership, places the leaders in a relationship of equality and symbiosis with the group, as far as the adoption and application of decisions is concerned. This leadership model is opposite to that of traditional leadership, characterized chiefly by a distance between the leader and the followers and by a centralization of decision-making power–at least as far as key decisions are concerned.

The leadership development that occurred in the four stages of the Casalta project sheds light on a number of interesting issues. In the first place, the meaning of leadership is elaborated in the course of the experience's development. Participatory leadership at the project's outset was defined according to the context at that time. But thereafter the participants, due to the imposition of other leaders by the government authorities, experienced an opposing–and less participatory–style of leadership. The resulting contrast provided them with an opportunity to compare the premises on which both leadership styles are based, whose result, given the inferiority of the imposed leadership, was the community's restoration of the leadership model it had previously developed. In the second place, and as a consequence thereof, the meaning of leadership elaborated by the group became a community value, to such an extent that forms of leadership inconsistent with this value are rejected by the community. In the third place, there is a close link between the quality of community participation and its leadership: as participation intensifies and its forms of expression evolve, the leadership must change as well, becoming more participatory, in order to be congruent with the ongoing changes of participation.

The similarity in the constructed nature of the meanings of organization and leadership, as argued earlier, and the direct relationship between both of them and the variations in community participation over time, suggest two important implications. First, the PC's organization and leadership are so closely intertwined that changes in one necessarily produce changes in the other. And second, both of them exert so much influence on the development of CP that they can validly be viewed as pillars of, or the foundation in which, the CP process is anchored.

LEADERSHIP IN FORMAL ORGANIZATIONS AND VOLUNTARY ORGANIZATIONS

Still another striking aspect of leadership in Casalta is the close link that comes into being between the leaders and the other members of the group, which stands in sharp contrast to the way leaders and followers interact in most formal organizations.

In those organizations, according to authors like Munene (1997), the leader is responsible for defining the events that occur in the organization; the leader provides the meaning expected to be shared by the followers. Accordingly, the leader does not take part in the implementation of decisions; that is the administrator's task. This approach circumscribes the creation of meanings in the organization to an individual act or that of a small elite, in whom the capacity for defining the organization's mission is vested. Participation is relegated to the application of decisions and kept separate from the leadership process.

Attempts have been made to overcome the leadership-participation dilemma present in the preceding definition, through proposals for integrating the two processes. According to Sagie and Koslowsky (1996), one of the proposed avenues for doing so makes a distinction between strategic and tactical decisions, as a way of including the organization's leadership or direction, and participation in decision making, in two distinct phases. Strategic decisions are those concerning the definition of the organization's direction of change, while tactical decisions refer to the means of implementing that change; in other words, they are tactics because they are decisions on the timing, form, and space in which the organization's change should be pursued.

The leaders or top management are the people directly involved in defining the organization's mission or ultimate ends, and they are the ones responsible for making the strategic decisions. For that reason, as Sagie and Koslowsky (1996) likewise point out, they are the appropriate human resources for structuring change during the uncertainty or turbulence that may occur while the organization is being restructured. Tactical decisions, on the other hand, are made with participation by the employees, since they are the people most familiar with the actions to be taken to implement the policies adopted at the higher level.

Another option described by Sagie (1997) conceives change in organizations as being composed of a decision phase followed by an execution phase. Participation and leadership are involved in both, but then the execution of the decisions is under the leadership's responsibility.

In these two conceptions there is no attempt to overcome the leadership-participation gap; the separation between the two processes persists. In the first option participation is restricted to the tactical decision sphere, while in the second it is minimized in the execution phase. What is more, these proposals are not valid alternatives for participatory community organizations, which have an entirely different form of operation. To begin with, there is no separation between leaders who take part in strategic decision making and other members who participate in tactical decisions; nor is there any such separation between decision making and execution. Furthermore, these organizations are often unable to clearly distinguish between strategic and tactical decisions, because the emergence of certain basic needs, in a context of meager opportunities to satisfy them, imposes a certain simultaneity on the decision-making process. Hence, in such situations the community may not wait long enough to first define its ends and then determine the ways in which it will achieve them; under pressure from the circumstances, tactical decisions may be executed in the midst of the decision-making process. To illustrate, while the Casalta community was busy defining the type of housing its members wanted, they illegally occupied the land on which the housing they were struggling to define would later be built.

To sum up, participatory action, by its very nature, requires the decisions made and the means adopted for their execution to be collective decisions; that is why the leadership-participation relationship is described as diluted. But this does not mean that the status of leader in a participatory process is insignificant. Quite the contrary, leadership is required, as is attested to by the participants of Casalta, but in a facilitating function that Sagie (1997) calls framework-substance. Leadership in the participatory decision-making model is called upon to moderate the production of ideas and formulate problems at a given time, since these are products on the basis of which it is then necessary to decide or create the substance of the decisions. But that substance is a collective function, as is implementation thereof, with no distance between leaders and led.

CONCLUSIONS

Community organization and leadership are two conditions of key importance for the continuity of CP, which are interlinked in view of the requirement for congruence between them. That is to say that community organization under a participatory-democratic model must be accompanied by a leadership of the same kind, to ensure the community's internal coherence. Furthermore, organization and leadership are two conditions that play a key role in the formation and scope of the project's goal and in the performance of actions that lower the cost of participation. The definition and achievement of the goal, however, also depend on the kind of support provided by external entities and the cost of participation for the community.

PROPOSITIONS

We suggest the following two proposals to promote continuity of community participation.

Relating to Community Organization

It has often been said that a community's organizational model develops in accordance with the participatory "nature" of the particular project on which the community embarks, as well as its equally participatory leadership. Two basic requirements that must be met by a participatory community's organization are that it be democratic and participatory as defined earlier. Based on these values, the organization can take different forms as circumstances warrant, but whatever model is chosen, it must incorporate mechanisms that regulate the balance between community participation and sectoral participation. In addition, community organizations must be viewed as what Katz and Khan (1966) describe as open organizations, meaning organizations existing in an interdependent relationship with their external environment. Hence, action strategies must be formulated to ensure their synergetic capability or their ability to attract and retain a variety of resources conducive to the achievement of their goal.

Relating to Leadership

Participatory leadership must have a profile in which the leader's visibility and accessibility are his or her outstanding characteristics, along with his or her expertise in taking initiatives, generating ideas, motivating people and stimulating communication in and with the community, and developing a kind of relationship that makes leadership a permanently shared condition. In this respect, training for leaders in community participation must focus on inducing them to think of themselves as articulators of the group's ideas, in permanent communication with its members, so that each party can generate feedback for the other during the participation process.

NOTES

1. All quotes of participants used in this article were gathered within the Casalta Project.
2. A more detailed description of the research design is found in Sánchez (2000).

REFERENCES

Chavis, D. M. Newbrough, J. R. (1986). The meaning of "community" in community psychology. *Journal of Community Psychology, 14*, 335-340.
Chinoy, E. (1968). *Introducción a la sociología*. Buenos Aires: Paidós.
Durham, H. W. (1986). Commentary. The community today: Place or process. *Journal of Community Psychology, 14*, 399-404.
Heller, K. (1989). The return to community. *American Journal of Community Psychology, 17*, 1-15.
Hubert, R. P. (1996). *La definición de comunidad: Una segunda mirada*. Unpublished manuscript.
Hunter, A. & Riger, S. C. (1986). The meaning of community in community mental health. *Journal of Community Psychology, 14*, 55-71.

Katz, D. & Khan, R. L. (1966). *The psychology of organizations*. New York: John Wiley & Sons.

Kieffer, C. (1984). Citizen empowerment: A developmental perspective. *Prevention in Human Services, 3*, 9-36.

McMillan, D. W. & Chavis, D. M. (1986). Sense of community: A definition and theory. *Journal of Community Psychology, 4*, 6-23.

Montero, M. (1998). La comunidad como objetivo y sujeto de la acción social. In A. Martín González (Ed.), *Psicología comunitaria: Fundamentos y aplicaciones* (210-222). Madrid, Spain: Síntesis.

Moreno, A. (1996). La psicología comunitaria en la realidad popular venezolana. *Heterotopia, 1*, 8-23.

Munene, J. C. (1997). On leaders, leaders-managers, managers, and participation. *Applied Psychology: An International Review, 46*, 427-430.

Pozas, A. R. (1964). *El desarrollo de la comunidad*. México: UNAM.

Sagie, A. (1997). Leader direction and employee participation in decision making: Contradictory or compatible practices? *Applied Psychology: An International Review, 46*, 387-452.

Sagie, A. & Koslowsky, M. (1996). Decision type, organizational control, and acceptance of change: An integrative approach to participative decision making. *Applied Psychology: An International Review, 45*, 85-92.

Sánchez, E. (2000). *Todos con La Esperanza: La continuidad de la participación comunitaria*. Caracas: Comisión de Estudios de Postgrado de la Facultad de Humanidades y Educación, UCV

Moral Dilemmas of Community Leaders and Sense of Community

Levy Farías
Gloria Perdomo

Universidad Central de Venezuela

SUMMARY. This paper draws on Kohlberg's theory of moral development, and on an empirical research conducted with leaders (two women, two men) in Venezuelan urban working-class communities. The leaders were repeatedly interviewed during a two-year period, about their experiences leading their communities. Those narratives were analyzed and discussed with them. Based on these grounds, two interrelated products were constructed: (1) Three moral dilemmas to be used in educational discussions with community leaders such as members of organized community groups; civic volunteers, officers from non-governmental organizations working with communities, and (2) A developmental approach to the sense of community in urban working-class communities. Finally, it argues about the need of balancing the current approaches of moral development, through a stronger emphasis on the community dimensions of that sense and its consequences on leadership. *[Article copies available for a fee from The Haworth Document Delivery Service: 1-800-HAWORTH. E-mail address: <docdelivery@haworthpress.com> Website: <http://www. HaworthPress.com> © 2004 by The Haworth Press, Inc. All rights reserved.]*

Address correspondence to: Levy Farías, Callejón Machado, Edif. Romeo, Piso 11, Apto. 114. Urb. El Paraíso. Caracas, 1021,Venezuela (E-mail: levyfdk@telcel.net).

The authors are indebted to Aracelis Maldonado for the translation and adaptation into English of the moral dilemmas.

[Haworth co-indexing entry note]: "Moral Dilemmas of Community Leaders and Sense of Community." Farías, Levy, and Gloria Perdomo. Co-published simultaneously in *Journal of Prevention & Intervention in the Community* (The Haworth Press, Inc.) Vol. 27, No. 1, 2004, pp. 25-37; and: *Leadership and Organization for Community Prevention and Intervention in Venezuela* (ed: Maritza Montero) The Haworth Press, Inc., 2004, pp. 25-37. Single or multiple copies of this article are available for a fee from The Haworth Document Delivery Service [1-800-HAWORTH, 9:00 a.m. - 5:00 p.m. (EST). E-mail address: docdelivery@ haworthpress.com].

http://www.haworthpress.com/web/JPIC
© 2004 by The Haworth Press, Inc. All rights reserved.
Digital Object Identifier: 10.1300/J005v27n01_03

KEYWORDS. Moral development, community leadership, sense of community, moral dilemmas

Moral wisdom, no doubt, is a social matter. Historical reports show that in the exceptional cases when an isolated child has managed to survive by herself or himself, s(he) has done so as a small beast, not as a true human being. On the other hand, figures such as Buddha, Thoreau or Gandhi demonstrate that moral advancement has also an undeniable individual component. It is not an easy task to study moral or ethical phenomena giving the due weight to its social and personal dimensions.

In general terms, seeking that equilibrium involves some ancient and complex debates, as discussed by Rubio (1996), Haste (1996), and many other authors (e.g., Lind, Hartmann and Wakenhut, 1985). But it is not the purpose of this paper to delve into the political or philosophical grounds of this discussion. Here we will present some tools and ideas that may be useful for researchers of collective moral development and for community workers or any practitioner or activist committed with such general values as democracy, justice, peace or solidarity.

These tools and ideas are based, in the first place, on theoretical approaches usually labeled as constructivist, cognitive-developmental or neopiagetian–mostly Kohlberg's theory of moral development, and in second place, on our research and professional experience with Venezuelan, urban, working-class communities (Farías, 1994, 2001; Perdomo, 1998, 2002). So, what we pretend to do here is to link an approach frequently accused of being highly individualistic with a culture historically characterized by its sense of community, collective solidarity–or in Spanish, by the value of *"convivencia"* (roughly translated as living together as a collective body).

KOHLBERG'S CONTRIBUTION TO COMMUNITY DEVELOPMENT: A BRIDGE TOO FAR?

The moral development theory proposed by Lawrence Kohlberg is generally recognized as one of the major landmarks in the psychosocial study of morality, but it also has been criticized for exaggerating the cognitive and individual processes involved in moral behavior. Certainly, the first decades of Kohlberg's work were deeply marked by those biases. But gradually, and especially after the energetic critics of a former associate, Carol Gilligan (1982), Kohlberg acknowledged the need of paying more attention to affective and group factors, and took part in several educational projects that gave shape to the "Just Community" Approach to Moral Education (Kohlberg, Power and Higgins, 1989/1997).

This turn represents an important advance, but one that needs to be consolidated, extending his scope from the alternative High Schools in which it was generated, to a wider range of groups or institutions. Indeed, even the core of Kohlberg's theory–the six stages of personal moral development–needs a major reformulation in order to overcome its individualistic slant. This was argued some time ago by Snarey, who–after reviewing 45 studies of moral development carried out in 27 countries– concluded that:

> Although strongly supportive of the stage structures currently identified, these findings also indicated that other *values, such as collective solidarity, that are commonly stressed in either traditional folk cultures or in working-class communities, are missing from the theory's explication* and the scoring manual's examples of reasoning at the higher stages. (Snarey, 1985: 226; emphasis added)

In other words, here we have an important theoretical gap that requires collaboration between developmental and community psychologists. And not only for the advantage of the former, because as we will try to show, this cooperation also may render educational materials useful in social or educative interventions.

SOME FREQUENT MORAL DILEMMAS OF COMMUNITY LEADERS

One of the most distinctive features of Kohlberg's theory is the use of hypothetical moral dilemmas: fictional situations in which the rights or duties of an individual conflict with the rights or duties of some other persons, forcing the interviewee (or the reader) to go beyond moral clichés, reasoning his way out of the dilemma. Asking insistently *why* the subject favors one of the given options or values, the researcher tries to overlook the content of the answer, focusing instead upon its structure or moral logic.

The "Heinz's dilemma," for example, surely the best known of these brief stories, presents to the reader the case of a man whose wife is going to die if she does not receive a new but very expensive drug. The dilemma and the subsequent questions discard the possibility of getting a loan, of persuading the greedy inventor of the drug to lower the price, etc. Thus the interviewee is forced to choose one of only two options available: steal the drug to save his wife, or let her die out of respect for the law. In essence, the dilemma opposes the value of a human life against the value of the property rights (for a summary of the moral dilemma's design and discussion techniques see Scharf, McCoy and Ross, 1979; or Hersh, Reimer and Paolitto, 1979).

As part of a measurement technique, the validity of this kind of dilemma is controversial, and some authors encourage wider or less artificial approaches, in order to describe and analyze the moral dilemmas that people actually experience in their lives. Johnston (1988), for example, has adapted some Aesop's fables, in order to explore not only how people solve certain dilemmas, but also how they construct them, when the situation admits diverse interpretations.

However, psychometric conundrums apart, it is clear that the systematic discussion of hypothetical moral dilemmas has beneficial–although moderate–effects on the moral reasoning of the participants. Having proved the shortcomings of an educational effort whose main or only strategy was the discussion of moral dilemmas, Kohlberg and his associates turned their attention to the moral atmosphere or justice structure of institutions (Power and Reimer, 1978).

Nevertheless, this does not imply that the discussion of moral dilemmas should be discarded. What is needed is attainment of an optimal distance regarding the actual moral conflicts in the life of the participants. Because the sort of reflection that is intended necessarily requires some degree of detachment, some cooling down of the passions may be involved. But the reflection will not arise if the examined situation looks too remote or farfetched. If the technique is going to have a reasonable probability of success it must challenge, somehow, the participant's usual thinking patterns.

From this point of view, the daily work and the studies of community psychologists represent a great deal of raw material that may be poured, for educational or civic purposes, in the form of hypothetical moral dilemmas. Qualitative studies tend to highlight the individual and community conflicts that usually arise in a given culture. The examples we present here were derived mainly from five life-stories of community leaders of Caracas working-class communities (Farías, 1994; 2001).

However, we think they depict some typical moral problems of any person who commits herself/himself to the common good of his neighborhood. So, these texts may be useful when working on adult education, with community leaders, voluntary social workers, non-governmental organizations, and the like.

Of course, these stories may be further tailored to the specific characteristics or situations of the participants. But setting aside the "literary" aspects, Dilemma 'A' (Box 1) evokes the frequent opposition between the feelings or experiences that drive some people to community or voluntary work, and the sacrifices that this kind of labor usually requires on the personal sphere. Dilemma 'B' (Box 2) poses the eternal questions of ends justifying means or the tension between ethics and politics, applied to what Sánchez (2000) sees as the central problem of social participation: how to maintain its continuity. While Dilemma 'C' (Box 3) invites reflection about the not-always-easy choice between two kinds of response to social problems: the paternalist, charitable but disempowering ones, and those that seek the initiative, self-organization or empowerment of the community.

Please note that these dilemmas are not aimed at a general audience. They are not intended for using with very selfish people or for counteracting the so-called "not in my backyard" syndrome. There are theoreti-

---

BOX 1
Dilemma A: So much for our homes!!!

José is a very hard-working person, permanently concerned about his community. But, even though he has been trying for years to mobilize his neighbors in order to solve many of their most urgent problems, very few people support or even hear him. Therefore, almost nothing has been achieved. During the last weeks, rumor has it that a shopping mall is going to be built exactly where they live. In order to do that, the government would have to tear down their homes. They would be relocated to some other place out of town, and they will receive a very low indemnification for their homes. During the first few days everything was just a rumor. But lately, in the local newspapers and TV stations, there have been a couple of stories regarding the construction of the shopping mall. Everybody in the neighborhood is just afraid! Nobody knows for sure when their properties will be torn down. Due to some contacts of José at the Mayor's office, he has been able to find out that everything is just an unfortunate misunderstanding, and there is really nothing to fear. Nevertheless, instead of calming down the neighbors with this great news, José has told them that the shopping mall is going to be built, no matter what. He is not doing this because he is mean or evil. He just feels that otherwise his neighbors will never learn how to organize themselves in order to deal with their problems.

At times, José has doubts about what he is doing, and feels guilty about lying to his neighbors, just like any other dishonest politician would do. But, when he sees his usually indifferent and careless neighbors now coming to meetings and working together, he forgets all remorse. He just keeps on spreading the bad news around.

Supposing that you were José... Would you do the same thing? Is it right to act in that way? Why?

BOX 2

Dilemma B: "You choose: The community or me."

Esteban is a young married man. Although he has been married for only two years, his wife, Evelyn, has already asked him for a divorce. He is not a womanizer, a drunkard or a wife beater, but he is late every night. Esteban loves Evelyn very much, but he is also the President of his Community's Board.

Lately the community has gone through some tough times. Besides the usual lack of water, trash all scattered around, and schools falling apart, they had to deal with a landslide that took some houses down, and several shootings that resulted in three people dead, and some wounded.

Since they got married, Evelyn knew about Esteban's involvement with his community. She used to admire him for that, but she never wanted to get too involved. Evelyn just wants to have kids, and a home of her own, since she is now living at her mother-in-law's. Evelyn is mostly annoyed, because Esteban is not getting any money for all the work he does for the community. Even worse, it is difficult for Esteban to find, let alone keep, a job, because every time his neighborhood is in trouble, he runs out to solve it. And with her job as a receptionist, Evelyn does not get enough money for the two of them.

On his part, Esteban recognizes that he has neglected his family duties, but he is also hurt. He thinks Evelyn does not understand him, and that it is unfair of her to make him choose between her and the community. Therefore, although he still is in love with her, he has started to think maybe it is better to get divorced.

Who is right? Should they get divorced? Should any of them change their attitude? Why?

BOX 3

Dilemma C: "Why me?"

Marisol is the "all time president" of her neighborhood association. At least, that is the way her friends call her, since she has been at that post for years, while nobody else wants to be elected. Not even the rest of the members do the job as they should. She works usually by herself, getting almost no help from anybody else.

It is only when imminent problems come up (like a broken pipe, or a serious landslide) that the rest of her neighbors recall the existence of the communal association, and run to Marisol for help. But she has had it! Marisol is so tired she is about to quit. Maybe when her neighbors have nobody to help them, they will have to organize themselves and grow up as a true community.

Nevertheless, her resignation does not seem possible just yet. "Who is going to take care of our elderly people? And who would keep our teenagers away from drugs, and who would fight so our infants get a kindergarten to go to?" These are all situations Marisol can not stop thinking about. Her conscience troubles her so much that she can't even sleep at night!

Marisol just does not know what to do! She constantly asks herself: Why does it have to be always me taking care of all our problems? But sometimes she wonders: If I do not take care of everything, who will?

What should one do in this case? If you were Marisol, what would you do? Why?

---

cal reasons to expect that, when reading the stories, the highly individualistic person will not see any dilemma at all. But we believe that in groups with at least some degree of receptivity to community efforts, and two or three incipient leaders, these kinds of materials may contribute to the moral development of both individuals and groups.

COMMUNITY SENSE:
A DEVELOPMENTAL SCHEME

Among the numerous contributions of the "Just Community" approach, there are several schemes of development that show how, working with the staff of some experimental or alternative high schools, researchers have been able to promote diverse expressions of collective moral development (Power and Makogon, 1995). One of those schemes, in particular, describes the observed evolution of the sense of community a process that comprehends five levels or degrees: (0) Rejection; (1) Instrumental Extrinsic; (2) Enthusiastic Identification; (3) Spontaneous Community; and (4) Normative Community (Kohlberg, Power and Higgins, 1997: 136).

May this sequence be used to understand or evaluate moral development in other kinds of communities? We believe so, but of course with some adjustments or extensions. Indeed, here we will try to adapt these levels to the social context of urban, working-class Latin-American communities. This will require modification of, mostly, the beginning and end of the developmental sequence.

The first level needs to be expanded or emphasized, because the Kohlbergnian approach characterizes it as an absence of communal notions or feelings, rather than a genuine or strong rejection. And to live in a *barrio* or Latin American slum generally does not imply an indifferent or disinterested attitude, but many intense and unavoidable experiences. Experiences of being discriminated against, oppressed, or excluded from society. Experiences embedded in a moral atmosphere that sets aside the normal, decent or "true" persons, from the "marginal" or supposedly worthless ones.

That's why some authors have used the term invisibility for describing the sociocultural status of black, Native American or poor Latin-American communities (Ontiveros & De Freitas, 1996: 133). The psychological counterpart of this invisibility may be illustrated through the testimony of Lourdes Pérez, a Venezuelan community leader, who was not aware that she lived in a slum, until the age of fifteen. It was only when she started to do some voluntary religious social work that Lourdes had that hard insight:

> Then I began to know what is to live in the slum [barrio], because I had not much contact with that. My life was mostly my home, and the factory. That is, . . . both things. At that moment I began to understand a bit, or to learn a bit more about the life in the slum, *and to realize that I also live in a slum! It is not . . . not easy, you know?*

I begin to realize this going to "Agua de maíz," more to those
slums [. . .] of the zone in which the factory was, *I realized that I
also live in a slum.* (Farías, 2001: 12; emphasis added)

About the intermediate levels, it seems to us that they don't require
major adjustments, but only identification of expressions equivalent to
those observed by Kohlberg and his disciples. In this sense, we think
that the best example of an *instrumental* sense of community is given by
the way in which some barrios are named. Because in our low income
communities, some communities give themselves traditional or geographic identifications, taking the name of historical figures or allegori-
cal dates ("Andrés Eloy Blanco," "January 23d," etc.); and quite a few
name themselves after the ruling President, the State Governor, or even
the name of the President's mistress! That is more frequent in those barrios surged through the *invasion* or illegal seizure of public or vacant
lands, where people do it hoping that in exchange, the person or the politician who receives the homage will provide his approval and protection or facilitate the reception of some sort of benefits: sewers, the
pavement of the street, electric power, etc.

Enthusiastic and Spontaneous levels are both characterized by a positive, intrinsic, but mainly affective sense of community. The difference
is that in the first of these phases the *esprit de corps* manifests itself only
on certain special occasions (like sportive games, holidays, etc.); and in
the second one is a rather stable or enduring attitude. Thus, in our view,
they may be fused together, and are surely a quite common phenomenon. Consider, for example, a testimony from Barrio La Ronda, in Ec-
uador: "Nowadays, one lives for living, and that's all. People only get
motivated at the Quito's holidays, *the city holidays is the only moment
of real unity*" (Bolívar, 1995: 49-50; emphasis added).

Now, as usually happens with evolutive schemata, the higher stages
are tougher, because they condense in themselves the rationale of the
whole sequence. On the other hand, it is pretty obvious that the focus on
high schools as context for dilemmas, no matter how democratic they
may be, simplifies too much the analysis of collective moral development, and over all, its political dimensions. In schools, a certain degree
of social innovation is usually tolerated. Instead, adult or "real" communities tend to behave in pretty conventional terms, unless urgent needs
or external threats prompt them to unify and mobilize themselves. In
most cases, however, once the urgencies are met or the menaces are
coped with, the mobilization decays and the sense of community weakens.

So, it seems reasonable to consider, as a working hypothesis, two final levels of this notion: one characterized by the temporary strengthening of the group's cohesion, in response to acute needs or external threats, in other words, a *vindicating*, but mainly defensive or reactive community sense; and a last–proactive–level characterized by a collective identification that, overcoming the ups and downs of community life, manages to affirm its distinctive social profile, on enduring, *institutional* grounds (compare with the "institutional" stage of self-development described by Kegan, 1982).

These higher levels surely imply diverse kinds of achievements or efforts: an affective bond to the land or territory; an affirmation of the historical or cultural features that integrates the community within the country, while simultaneously differentiating it from neighbor communities; etc. But for brevity's sake we will focus our attention on what seems to be the most troublesome or ambiguous point: the legal or political status of the community.

At this point, we believe that the Kohlberg approach is prone to emphasize, in a rather naive fashion, the systematic or rational character of legal systems, a flaw that could lead to overlooking the usual conflicts between the collective advancement of small or medium scale communities, and the metropolitan or national laws.

Consider, for instance, the struggle against the Venezuelan State of "La Morán" (a Caracas working-class community), during the years 1974-1983. In this case, documented and analyzed by Giulietta Fadda (1990), the inhabitants organized themselves against the governmental plans to dispossess them of their houses, paying them an extremely low indemnification. Thus, they had several vindicating successes. However, so to speak, those triumphant battles led them to the loss of the war. The government was forced to compensate the residents with new and more or less comfortable apartments, but shrewdly relocating the families in different suburbs or buildings, the state provoked the weakening, and in the long run the complete extinction, of what was once a vigorous social movement (Fadda, 1990: 198-199).[1]

A second case also dated in the seventies, but with a different outcome, is the "Monterrey's possessors' movement," documented and analyzed by Castells (1981). This movement, that involved 100,000 persons grouped in 26 highly organized "colonies" (equivalent to barrios), took possession of governmental lands and resisted several repressive attempts by the Mexican state. But when the government reluctantly accepted to legally recognize the occupation of the lands, the movement refused what, apparently, was their dearest objective. This paradoxical refusal had to do, to some extent, with the high and prolonged payments required for the land. But it had to do mostly with the political consequences of the agreement. The community leaders were aware that accepting a legal and individual relationship with the state implied fragmentation of the movement,

> thus, in order to preserve their solidarity, their cohesion, their strength, that is, their *only weapons*, the possessors rejected the legal regularization that had been repeatedly offered to them by the authorities, and proceeded to expulse from the colonies all those inhabitants who had accepted the State titles. (Castells, 1981: 181)

All this happened in the context of a sharp ideological conflict: the organization of the colonies included "Honor and Justice Committees," "Defense and Vigilance" teams, feminine and infantile "Leagues," and "Activist's Brigades" in charge of the cultural activities of the "Red Sundays." Alcohol and prostitution were forbidden within the communities, and some colonies decided collectively to reject the installation of electricity, in order to prevent TV's "ideological contamination." Besides, the movement adopted a strategy of "Just causes support," in favor of other collective or individual conflicts. In 1976, when the Castells' study finished, the movement had split into two rival factions, and faced serious inner conflicts.

A third and last case worthy of attention, although it involves a smaller population, is the experience of "Los Erasos" (a Caracas working-class community) in delinquency prevention. This experience, that took place in the nineties, had as a culminating moment the signing, by a group of Venezuelan juvenile delinquents, of a "Commitment Act" that, among other things, declared:

1. We assume the commitment of not executing, and avoiding in the future, the perpetration of criminal acts, transgressions and other deeds violating the Republic's Laws. . . .
4. We assume the commitment of our integration to civic life, obeying its Laws and coexistence rules; expecting in the same way, that the society and its institutions accept our commitment and offer us a better opportunity, through jobs, enabling us to work in a honest and peaceful way (Farías, 1994: 321).

So, it should be clear that the institutional development of the community encompasses much more than legal or bureaucratic advances. Or in other words, that the institutional level is not always reached thanks to the law, but sometimes in spite of the law.

In sum, trying to go beyond the particular instances, Box 4 offers our views about the development of a sense of community, a scheme that requires two important caveats. First, please note that all these levels are developmental in a very mild sense; they should not be taken as stages in a strict, Piagetian sense. They are rather ideal types, hierarchically organized, to be used within certain sociocultural contexts. Second, we are not claiming that these levels are enough for evaluating thoroughly the moral development of a collectivity. It should be obvious that several other factors, as the kind of leadership, the degree of equity existent within the community, the values embraced, etc., are also relevant.

COMMUNITY SOLUTIONS FOR INDIVIDUAL DILEMMAS?

As a final point, we wish to comment on a remarkable coincidence. Almost a decade before Kohlberg began to use the Heinz's dilemma, a Mexican filmmaker, Emilio "Indio" Fernández, had already posed the same moral situation in his movie *La bienamada* [She, the beloved one] (1951). Of course, some details differ: the man's name is Antonio, not Heinz, and the money is needed for an operation, not for a drug. But the dilemma is strikingly similar: the wife's life vs. the law. Even the malady is the same–cancer. However, despite the same departure point, the movie and the psychological test run along different lines.

BOX 4
Sense of community levels

A. *"Invisibility" or rejection.* The feeling of belonging to the community is seen as pejorative and shameful. The individual avoids or denies his belonging to the community.
B. *Extrinsic instrumental.* The individual values the community only in terms of territoriality or in reference with his most basic needs, cutting out its character as a social group ("The weather is nice here." "It's close to my work." "There's a dispensary.").
C. *Spontaneous identification.* The community is valued intrinsically, but mainly in affective terms. This may occur during special occasions (sports events, religious festivities), or in a rather stable basis ("We are all friends," "We know each other since we were kids," etc.).
D. *Vindicating identification.* The community is valued intrinsically, during relatively long periods of time, due to its efficacy or usefulness for claiming the solution to acute collective problems, or for tackling menaces like evictions, robberies, drug-problems, and the like.
E. *Institutional identification.* The community is positively valued as a social entity greater than the sum of its present dwellings, inhabitants or friendly relationships. This kind of identification encompasses, as main axes:

- The effective domain of a territory, and a positive evaluation of it.
- The account of the community's historical and cultural distinctive physiognomy.
- The struggle for a legal definition–or redefinition–of the community.

The Kohlberg test does not take into account either accidental outcomes, or community interventions. In the movie, Antonio first tries to steal the money armed with a knife, but being a school teacher, he proves unfit for the task and only gets hurt. Then he steals the school's savings, the money that pupils and their parents had amassed cent by cent. So he is able to pay for the costly operation, but nevertheless his wife dies, after giving birth to a girl. Once the theft is discovered, Antonio is sent to jail, amidst a big scandal. But later, when the school's community learns about the sad circumstances that led the poor man to break the law, they decide to give him the money as a present, and demand of the authorities his liberation.

Does all this mean anything? Maybe if Kohlberg would have seen the movie, it would have helped him to achieve a better understanding of the moral domain and its collective dimensions. Or maybe not. Whatever the case, nowadays, in moral development studies persists an individualistic bias that must be counteracted, not only out of respect for feminine morality (Gilligan, 1982), or for achieving wider, cross-cultural understandings, but also for sheer practical reasons. At least for us, writing from a country usually considered as rich, due to its huge oil reserves, but that, as we write this, is importing gasoline and at the brink of a civil war, it is pretty obvious that social scientists could and should do more to elucidate the complex and sometimes paradoxical relations between the individual and the community dimensions of moral development.

NOTE

1. Nevertheless, La Moran recovered from that blow, and in the last eight years its members have embarked on a co-managed community project, so far successful.

REFERENCES

Bolívar, T. (1995). *Hacedores de ciudad* [City makers]. Caracas,Venezuela: Universidad Central de Venezuela/Fundación Polar/Consejo Nacional de la Vivienda.

Castells, M. (1981). *Crisis urbana y cambio social* [Urban crisis and social change]. Madrid, Spain: Siglo XXI.

Fadda Cori, G. (1990). *La participación política como encuentro: Discurso político y praxis urbana* [Political participation as encounter: Political discourse and urban praxis]. Caracas, Venezuela: Acta Científica Venezolana/Universidad Central de Venezuela.

Farías, L. (1994). El papel de las organizaciones vecinales en el control y prevención de la delincuencia: Un testimonio desde 'Los Erasos' [The role of neighborhood organizations in the control and prevention of delinquency: A testimony from 'Los Erasos'] *Politeia* (17), 283-323.

Farías, L. (2001). *Del bien común como problema íntimo* [On common good as an intimate problem]. Ph.D. dissertation. Caracas, Venezuela: Universidad Central de Venezuela.

Gilligan, C., Ward, J.C. & McLean Taylor, J. (Eds.), *Mapping the Moral Domain*. Cambridge, USA: Harvard University Press.

Gilligan, C. (1982). *In a different voice*. Cambridge, USA: Harvard University Press.

Haste, H. (1996). Communitarianism and the Social Construction of Morality. *Journal of Moral Education, 25* (1), 47-55.

Hersh, R., Reimer, J., & Paolitto, D. (1979). *Promoting Moral Growth from Piaget to Kohlberg*. New York: Longman.

Kegan, R. (1982). *The evolving self* (Problem and Process in Human Development). Cambridge, USA: Harvard University Press.

Kohlberg, L., Power, F.C., & Higgins, A. (1997). *La educación moral según Lawrence Kohlberg*. Barcelona, Spain: Gedisa. [Originally published as: (1989). *Lawrence Kohlberg's Approach to Moral Education*, Columbia University Press].

Lind, Georg, H. H., & Wakenhut, R. (Eds.). (1985). *Moral Development and the Social Environment*. Chicago: Precedent.

Ontiveros, T. & De Freitas, J. (1996). Repensando el barrio: Papel del antropólogo en la rehabilitación de los espacios autoproducidos [Rethinking the slum: Role of the anthropologist in the rehabilitation of self-produced spaces]. In T. Bolívar & J. Baldó (Eds.), *La cuestión de los barrios* [The slums issue]. Caracas, Venezuela: Monte Avila–Fundación Polar–Universidad Central de Venezuela.

Perdomo, G. (1998). *Comprendiendo a la comunidad a través de la Investigación Acción Participativa* [Understanding the Community through Participatory Action-Research]. Caracas, Venezuela: Fundación Escuela de Gerencia Comunitaria.

Perdomo, G. (2002). Modos de actuar la corresponsabilidad entre los sectores empobrecidos y los poderes públicos [Modes of acting the corresponsibility between impoverished sectors and public agencies] *Iter, 27* 157-166.

Power, C. & Reimer, J. (1978). Moral atmosphere: An educational bridge between moral judgment and action. *New Directions for Child Development, 2*, 105-116.

Power, F. C. & Makogon, T. A. (1995). The Just Community Approach to Care. *Journal for a Just and Caring Education, 2*, 9-24.

Rubio Carracedo, J. (1996). *Educación moral, postmodernidad y democracia* [Moral education, postmodernity and democracy]. Madrid, Spain: Trotta.

Sánchez, E. (2000). *Todos con la "Esperanza." Continuidad de la participación comunitaria* [All of us are with "Hope." Continuity of community participation]. Caracas, Venezuela: Universidad Central de Venezuela.

Scharf, P., McCoy, W., & Ross, D. (1979). *Growing up moral: Dilemmas for the intermediate grades*. Minneapolis, USA: Winston Press.

Snarey, J. R. (1985). Cross-Cultural Universality of Social-Moral Development: A Critical Review of Kohlbergnian Research. *Psychological Bulletin, 97, 2,* 202-232.

Community Leaders:
Beyond Duty and Above Self-Contentedness

Maritza Montero

Universidad Central de Venezuela

SUMMARY. This paper presents the outcomes of ten years of community psychology practice in three low-income communities in the city of Caracas, and the way community leaders deal with the organization and relate to the persons that integrate their communities, as observed both by the author and some of her students, and colleagues. The general characteristics of community leadership and its participatory condition are discussed. Field notes, the leaders' interviews and narratives, and participant observation provided the data to be analyzed. Four modes of leadership are analyzed and illustrated with examples: The transformational leader; the narcissistic-seductive leaders in their positive and their negative expressions, and the altruistic leader. These categories are described, pointing out their assets and limitations. Finally, some tips on the relation between external agents working in the community and the community leaders are given. *[Article copies available for a fee from The Haworth Document Delivery Service: 1-800-HAWORTH. E-mail address: <docdelivery@haworthpress.com> Website: <http://www.HaworthPress.com> © 2004 by The Haworth Press, Inc. All rights reserved.]*

Address correspondence to: Maritza Montero, Apdo 80394. Prados del este. Caracas, 1080-A. Venezuela (E-mail: mmontero@reacciun.ve).

[Haworth co-indexing entry note]: "Community Leaders: Beyond Duty and Above Self-Contentedness." Montero, Maritza. Co-published simultaneously in *Journal of Prevention & Intervention in the Community* (The Haworth Press, Inc.) Vol. 27, No. 1, 2004, pp. 39-52; and: *Leadership and Organization for Community Prevention and Intervention in Venezuela* (ed: Maritza Montero) The Haworth Press, Inc., 2004, pp. 39-52. Single or multiple copies of this article are available for a fee from The Haworth Document Delivery Service [1-800-HAWORTH, 9:00 a.m. - 5:00 p.m. (EST). E-mail address: docdelivery@haworthpress.com].

http://www.haworthpress.com/web/JPIC
© 2004 by The Haworth Press, Inc. All rights reserved.
Digital Object Identifier: 10.1300/J005v27n01_04

KEYWORDS. Community leadership, transforming leaders, narcissistic-seductive leaders, altruistic leaders

This paper is based on the observation and reflection carried out during my practice and teaching of psychosocial community psychology concerning community leadership, a subject I have found difficult to grasp, sometimes exasperating, and full of surprises. I believe most community organisations and psychologists have had to lead with both the lack of community leaders, and the excesses of some community leaders, and every community psychologist knows how efficient and surprising can be community leaders. The reflections I want to share have been gathered at work with three community programmes in low income zones of the city of Caracas, Venezuela. The data were collected between 1992-2001 under the form of fieldwork notes, interviews, and group discussions carried out by myself (Montero, 1995) and by some of my undergraduate and graduate students (Farías, 2002), and research assistants (Domínguez, 2001). What I have done is to study the interviews and transcriptions of discussions looking for the narratives of leaders of those communities, referring to their conception of their task as conductors of community activities, and compare them with my own notes (another narrative), describing community working sessions, workshops, and assemblies where they had participated. And this is what I have learned and produced out of that process.

CHARACTERISTICS OF COMMUNITY LEADERSHIP

Perhaps the first point to be made clear is that community leadership shows some characteristics that differentiate it from the traditional perspective used to define leadership in general. It has been said, and it seems to be true for most leaders, that they work a lot more than any other member in the group, and it is also recognised that, as they are the most visible head in the group, they might end as being the scapegoats in case things end badly for the group; but it is also true that to lead a group, to give orders and exercise some power is something that many people seem to enjoy. But when we come to examine what happens in communities, many community leaders assume the task of conducting community groups in a very responsible way, knowing that it will be a tiring, exhausting and difficult one. And because of that many a time qualified people will not accept it. I have witnessed how some folks step in charge with a committed and responsible conviction, while considering it not exactly as forced labour, but very near it.

As we shall see later, community leadership covers a range of expressions that goes from civic sanctity to bordering on sanctified hypocrisy. Usually community leaders make themselves known during community meetings dealing with planning or carrying out some action; but sometimes leadership resides not only in the most verbal, but somehow in silent but very well respected people. These string-pulling, advice-giving, direction-pointers are not so easily detected, but their participation is precious and should not be left aside, especially since community leadership is mediated by participation.

THE PARTICIPATORY CHARACTER
OF COMMUNITY LEADERSHIP

Although every group does produce leaders, their acceptance by the rest of the members may be influenced by their capacity and quickness to produce answers and ways of solving problems; by their offer to do it; by their being known by the group members; by how much they trust them, and by the history of actions they have shared. When community action has a participatory character, directing the group is something that arises by consensus; plans and decisions are made by reflective discussions and the actions derived of those decisions are carried out by many members. In those cases leaders usually become very popular within the community, which sees them as engaged in the defence of the collective interest, and tends to be supportive of them.

Another characteristic has to be added: *complexity*, a condition shared by most processes studied by community psychology and social sciences in general. Other aspects, are to be highlighted: *necessity and inevitability*. This last aspect, in my experience, has to be contextually analysed. As said before, being a community leader is no easy task; it is very demanding. Community leaders in the low-income and slum neighbourhoods I have worked with have to put up with a never completely satisfied collective, ready to criticise, difficult to mobilise, enormously complex in its diversity and, because of a history of deceptions, unfulfilled promises, and scarcity, very much distrustful. Therefore, although they also know by experience the power of community action, they tend to wait and see the first achievements, and they tend to act when the goal is clear, attainable, and directly related to some benefit, for they also know the costs. They will not trust someone unless they have measured and known that person for a while, according to her deeds.

Hernández (1998), working with leaders in rural areas of the Venezuelan Andes, found that the leaders (women and men) evaluated their performance as such, as a function of: (1) having acquired the capacity to organise and direct, (2) being considered by the people in the community as models of active persons and as sources of information and opinion, (3) having a deep commitment with their communities. They also consider themselves as significant according to the goals achieved under their lead. These characteristics coincide with what leadership theories say: the active character of leaders; their being the visible head of the group; and having the task of representing the group before institutions and other groups.

But the most outstanding characteristic, derived of the democratic aspect of participation, is shown in the fact that, although talking about leaders means also talking about followers, a participatory community has the possibility for any member to express her/his point of view. And even though that does not always happen due to lack of interest or because some people agree with what is being carried out, delegating those in charge, a good community leader tries to obtain the opinion of all participants. And this is not an unreal conception, for concerned community leaders manage to find out (asking directly; also doing it in an indirect way; surveying, opening consulting periods). Their leadership depends on that sort of contact. The main characteristics of community leadership are shown in Box 1.

A woman leader in a slum in the Eastern part of the city of Caracas said about the so-called leaders, formally elected, that do not respond to the community needs, and whose leadership she, among others, had substituted:

BOX 1

Characteristics of community leadership
-Participatory.
-Democratic.
-Complex.
-Active.
-Generates and empowers commitment among the community members.
-Is assumed as a service.
-Provides models for action and sources of information for the community.
-Has a political character directed to construct collective welfare.

Here [in that community], the Neighbours Association is more like
. . . dictatorial. It seems to be hard for the people belonging to it, to
leave it. Years and years go by, and they keep self-electing themselves. Mrs. X, she lives across [the street], and Mr. Z, up there;
since I came [to live] here, that Mr. was the Board President, and
he still is. . . . He elects himself. (Farías, 2002: Vol. I, 65)

THE TRANSFORMATIONAL LEADERSHIP

During my community praxis working along with a diversity of community leaders I have been both awed and annoyed, while sharing responsibilities with those leaders has taught me a lot. The first thing that
positively impacted me is an extraordinary type of leadership produced
in circumstances characterised by their participatory orientation, that
could be considered as a *transformatory* or *transformational* leadership. This coincides with what Bass described under that denomination
in 1985. A leadership based on genuine and deep affection exchanged
between leaders and participants, energetic, producing effective work
and the corresponding motivation (see Box 2).

This, which could be considered as the positive epitome, is no ordinary leadership. It is not frequent, but it does exist. It can be defined by
the presence of a strong and intense affective component; by an energetic display of work, carried out not only by the leader, but also by the
other people in the group. It has an activating effect on the group and its
influence area. In some cases (Farías, 2000) that activity of the leaders
can be extraordinary. Moreover, transformational leaders develop strong
links with other community members, who even the less participatory
respond to with congeniality and affection.

R., a leader in a Caracas *barrio*, illustrates some of those qualities:

Since I was a child, I had this preoccupation to demonstrate [that it
is possible for] the community within a barrio to live well, if the
people work to ameliorate their living conditions, . . . living in a
barrio cannot mean [to get] a label, . . . the people there have to
work for the improvement of their community, and they should
personally improve, because to live in a barrio does not mean not
being able to go to college, not being able to find a job. (Farías,
2002: 116)

BOX 2
Transformational Leadership: Characteristics

- They motivate the people, mobilising and inducing them to carry out or to contribute in a more intense manner than what they had originally offered, or than had been expected.
- They try to foster and increase the participation of shy or detached individuals. In general, they try to increase the number of active members both in the organising core and in activities, engaging the largest possible number of people in the various tasks, distributing thus the efforts and developing commitment.
- They place the welfare of the communities and the organised groups within them above personal interests, stimulating community development.
- Together with active persons in the communities they induce changes in the needs hierarchy and re-define the needs felt, reflecting about the causes of specific problems. They foster a mobilisation of consciousness towards latent needs.
- They stress the rewarding character of community achievements for the people participating in them, and for other people in the community. They celebrate and enjoy community tasks.
- Their words and deeds become a model and an inspiration for other community participants, for other organised groups, and for the community as a whole.
- They try to intellectually stimulate both the participants in community activities and other people in the communities. They care for the personal development of participants.
- They have personal charm, and even charisma. They do not react to critics in a negative way. They are cheerful, caring, affectionate and open.
- They have a face-to-face relationship with each participant, communicating easily with people in the community, being concerned with their daily problems, attentively listening to them. They provide guidance and advice.
- They keep the people informed, so the activities of organised groups and the problems in the variety of groups and tendencies within a community are known by everyone. They try to make efforts and difficulties shared by all community members.
- They delegate responsibilities in other group members, fostering their development and best capacities.
- They are respectful of dissidence and ready to negotiate in order to join forces, without sacrificing the community welfare and goals.

R. is a leader who continuously motivates people to learn and also wants to learn more himself; he also finds joy in what he does: "What I do, that is what I enjoy" (Farías, 2002: 127); he is self-demanding; setting himself higher goals and looking for the best; carefully planning expenses and at the same time, experimenting with new ways to do things (Farías, 2002: 124-132).

Transformational leaders are one of the best assets in a community, but they are hard to find. The ordinary community leader is, as most human beings are, a mixture of good, average, and luckily, few bad traits. The interchange within a participatory community manages to get the best of the good and average, and to control or to reduce the negative effects of the bad or even to accept them as part of the package. But there are two types of leaders I would like to discuss specifically. I am referring to a type of charming, seductive, well-spoken leader, who is very devoted to some community causes, and at the same time the origin of some very negative situations. These leaders I have denominated as *narcissistic-seductive*, and they can be *positive* or *negative*.

THE POSITIVE NARCISSISTIC-SEDUCTIVE LEADER

This category could be considered as a *good* bad leader in the sense that they have a positive orientation towards the community. They usually arc kind, gentle, nice, full of good intentions, but their high amount of activity in the community's benefit is characterised, in a subtle and always gentle way, by blocking, in an indirect, suave, convincing and firm manner, any activity or idea not originated by them. This is someone leading with a great deal of sacrifice, enormously diligent, always looking for the community's benefit, but who may delay activities and plans because they do not fit in his idea of how things should be done. And because he is respected and loved by other community members, once again they will discuss decisions already approved, until they respond to what the leader wishes.

The cost of this is very high: It can arrest efforts, slowing them and making people lose motivation and become dispirited, things do not change (and usually community groups do not want to lose time), and participation begins to thin out. It is also high for the leader, for he/she becomes overloaded with work, because in his/her wish to control s(he) assumes or supervises more tasks than s(he) should and can carry out. Formally they delegate, but always keep charge. This shows they do not trust in other members' capacities, and although they do not make that manifest, that is the message their behaviour is transmitting.

This results in repeatedly carrying out certain chores, and even if they are well made, it means spending more energy than is necessary. At the same time, many other tasks that could have been made never take place, and in the end the participants' enthusiasm and initiative diminishes and they retire. People start to solely participate in specific actions, and the leader and a small group finish directing all the movement, very tired, overworked, loved by everyone, but at the same time solitary and criticised in low voice for not admitting new ideas and for excluding other possible participants. And although theirs is not the production of personal winnings (actually they invest much of their time and effort), this way of leading community work can be considered as narcissistic because their behaviour means they consider that no one can do things the way they do. No one loves the community better or more than they do. Nobody will sacrifice more than they do. They are the best.

THE NEGATIVE NARCISSISTIC-SEDUCTIVE LEADER

This denomination refers to a leader also very much attached to the community, very nice and agreeable, with explicit participatory interests, who loves and admires leading roles and leaders playing them, and who wants to be one of them and be admired and congratulated. Their motivation is then more egocentric and narcissistic than the previous type, and it is not mainly oriented by collective welfare, but by individualistic interests that he/she can satisfy by means of community work. Achieving community goals comes to be, then, a collective means to obtain an individual objective. This is the leader who appropriates other people's ideas without giving credit to their authors; or presents them as introduced by himself/herself. He/she reduces or diminishes other participants' intervention, subtly denying their abilities and creativity, while illuminating those self-attributed. He/she can lie, manipulate, and pile functions in order to increase his/her own importance. When presenting other people's activities or results he/she uses expressions such as "I rescued so and so," "I elevated so and so," "I am helping so and so," thus implying the limitations or weaknesses of those people. This may induce feelings of discapacity and helplessness or, in general, negative self-attributions in the participants, generating passivity, confirming then the image the leader is presenting of them. In that way, participation may decline or disappear, for a negative narcissistic-leader cannot ensure a lasting project (for an example, see Box 3).

Although this category of leaders can develop a lot of activity, its success does not last. People attend their call, but there are very few results because the leader is concerned with his own promotion, forgetting the collective welfare. They even can present as their own the work carried out by the group, in order to obtain prestige and support from institutions or agencies, without consulting with the community and the people involved. It is not easy for a community to get rid of this type of leader. When confronted, they give many excuses, trying if possible to blame whatever it is they are accused of on other participants. If their arguments are not convincing, they will accept the responsibility, but will

BOX 3

A negative narcissistic-seductive leader cannot ensure a lasting project. An example.
A community in Caracas has had for several years a small radio transmitter working twice a week to announce birthdays, deaths, vaccination campaigns, and other information useful for the community, plus popular music the days the clothes bazaar is open. Traditionally the ones in charge of the Radio are teen-agers. But as they grow and have to deal with high school, college studies, or get jobs, the group gets smaller and approximately every two years it disappears. Soon there will be a new one, very energetic, with new projects and programmes. W is a 36-38 year-old adult, assiduous collaborator of some community projects and social work in the zone. He decides to take in charge the Radio, whose last directing group has outgrown its directorship. He proposes the task to a small group of children (10-13 years old) and a couple of teen-agers. They are very enthusiastic and begin to plan their programmes. W initiates a successful campaign telling neighbours, visitors, and NGOs workers how he is "rescuing" those children lost in the barrio, how "he has inspired them" to do some "useful work," and how he has also "created" the Radio as a project to "recover children lost in the streets of the barrio." W's discourse constructs a narrative in which he is a creator figure and presents his young collaborators as children in danger, unable to do something useful by themselves, therefore lost or in the process of "getting lost." The children work hard at the beginning: they write the scripts for the programmes, they read what they had prepared, but W presented all the achievements as his own. A few months later the children stopped talking about their Radio experiences and dispersed. Actually, all the children have at least one responsible parent, go to school, belong to the special programmes being developed in the neighbourhood, and are neither "lost" nor in the process of becoming so. The children felt used, lost interest or grew tired of being ignored as participants and authors. The project was not theirs. And as he was left alone, W also got tired, but of doing the work all by himself.

try to save their status by appealing to their personal links with community members, or to their past participation, and adopting a humble and friendly attitude until the conflict wanes or is over. What makes them different from many other opportunistic people in other settings is that they are charming, they are seductive, they kiss and hug a lot, and they are not only accepted, but even liked by the very people they will try to use for their personal interests.

THE DIFFICULT ASPECTS OF COMMUNITY LEADERSHIP

As with any leadership, what can be found in the community is not exempt of certain problems such as the conflicts that can rise between personal interest of the leaders and the community collective interests. Also, the leader status and the desire to occupy it can give way to rivalries and struggles between members of the community aspiring to lead. This type of confrontation can be found in different settings (i.e., institutions, rural areas, sport teams). In fact, it is a problem that now and then comes up in any group, and actually what is important is the capacity of the community to cope with that situation, resolving the difficulty. If the community discusses it in a democratic way, with collective interests and goals in mind, it will come out strengthened.

The same can be said about the power clash between leaders within the same community. A community can have several leaders, according to the different projects being carried out within it and the different needs or problems to be solved. Sometimes objectives superpose or contradict one another, and that leads to confrontations between not only leaders, but also other participants.

Working with Venezuelan low-income communities, one can witness how their leaders have to attend to many, and very difficult, tasks. And also how, being the spokespersons of the organised groups within the community, they not only have the doors slammed in their faces, but also how they are blamed and chased; and even worse, how after achieving a specific goal, see how it is taken away or destroyed by someone with institutional power. These tremendous hurdles produce a sort of "burnout" in community leaders, conducive to excessive rotation of them. I have seen how very committed leaders complain about how much time from family and leisure they have to devote to community problems. Sometimes they become anxious when they think that there will not be other persons to efficiently replace them, so they will not be able to step down and take some rest. Because of this, in some communities there is much reluctance to fill the position (Hernández, 1998). In this case, collective needs invade the space and time of individual needs, and the price the leaders have to pay is very high: no time for their families, no time for their health, nor time for their personal projects. Besides, overworked leaders end up not being able to fulfil their duties in an adequate way. They are so tired, so nervous, so jumpy, they forget things, postpone meetings, arrive late or fail to appear, and feel miserable because of that. And as Hernández (1998) has registered: they have no time for reflection about what is happening around them.

And in community contexts, as in institutional, organisational, political or any other contexts, one can find community leaders that have been very successful in the past, and as they have become the leading reference for their community, they find themselves in a comfortable position, not challenging any more. So they begin to repeat the gestures that were previously successful, somehow creating a routine, ritualising the task and not caring to learn new things. When that style fails before an unexpected situation, those leaders have become an obstacle. Two things can happen: the people surrounding them, out of respect and affection, do not want to ask them to step aside, and abandon the task, losing motivation and commitment; or they just by-pass the old leader and some new leader assumes the chore. This is very hard for the old guard, and could have been avoided if the group had kept a system to alternate leaders. Too much rotation is bad, too little is sometimes worse, since everyone loses.

BEYOND DUTY–THE ALTRUISTIC LEADERS: A COMMUNITY PHENOMENON

There are ordinary leaders, those who begin with a lot of impulse; have some success; make some errors; correct them; establish a routine; get tired and then get substituted, or simply step out to leave place for new ideas. There are transformational leaders; and nice and obnoxious leaders both oriented by the conviction they can do better than others; some to protect and do good (good bad leaders); some to enjoy some power and be the centre of attention (bad good leaders). And there are extraordinary leaders. Leaders that go beyond duty. And they seem to be, at least in my experience, a community phenomenon, although surely they exist in other types of social relations. Those are the *altruistic leaders*, those whose lead of community activities goes over what is considered a good performance, exceeding what was expected and constituting a higher stage of ethics. That is, consideration and respect for others, represented not only by the collective of their community, but by the human condition. Saints? Neither do they consider themselves as such, nor do other people in their community see them in that way. Certainly they are respected, followed, and loved by many among their neighbours, fellows and friends, and they receive the admiration of external agents. They recognise their weaknesses and wrongs, and they confess their dislikes and nuisances. A life narrative of one such a leader interviewed by Farías (2002) gives an example of how they view their task (see Box 4).

Psychological Aspects Present in Altruistic Leaders

Altruistic leaders are convinced that their task as co-ordinators, conductors of community activities, is part of a collective movement in which they have a specific role, and they encourage and look for other people's participation. The tasks they have to carry out they see as part of

BOX 4

An altruistic leader speaks about his task.
I live all of this not as a job. Firstly, I have never felt this as a job. Of course, then with the family, with friends, with life itself... I, in a self-critical way, we could consider that as an error, couldn't I?. . . The other aspect is health. Sometimes I feel ill, or I have some health problem... Sometimes that is not a reason to interrupt my work. Then, that should not happen, one should have some rest . . . and I know I should go to the Doctor, and I do not visit the Doctor because I think this is more important. That's it: not feeling this situation as some kind of work. . . . I sleep on average between four and five hours. . . .I draw forces from love. I love to love. I feel good. . . . I have that feeling when I am with my family, with people, with children, with the community. . . . Some people get mad at me and become angry: "But, why do you always speak saying "We"? Why do you always speak in plural? . . . And it happens that the answer is easy and simple. When one has the moral support, that beautiful and handsome support, and the confidence of the people, that even when they are a few, they are valuable people, that have a lot of dignity, and they support your process, your. . . life action, that support already is part of the so-called "we"; because I am not alone, I do not feel alone. A Narrative. Farías (2002:231-232, 236).

a process of learning and teaching that gives them pleasure and is impassioned. It is regarded as their life task. They have feelings of love and they are very respectful of people in their community, and in general, all human beings (altruistic feelings).

What Farías (2002) and I also have observed in our community practice is that these altruistic leaders are characterised by *solidarity* with the people in their communities, expressed in the help they give, in sharing their joys and sorrows, in feelings and demonstrations of fraternity. And this solidarity is linked to their religiousness. Farías (2002) made four life narratives of community leaders (two men, two women), working along with them for several years. Two of those leaders I have known and worked with for at least six years, and one of the things that has impacted me most is the *deep religiousness* they show. Their belief in a superior Being is not expressed in formal or liturgical ways; it is part of their daily lives. They speak of God in the most natural way, as a presence by their side, as a source and as a force, as a beloved friend they completely trust. And that religiousness does not mean a fanatical attitude. Their beliefs do not necessarily express a specific cult, although some of them are Catholic.

Other characteristics they show are their *creativity* and *imagination* in the sense that they have what I may call a poetic conception of life, in the Greek sense of the word *poiesis*, meaning creative capacity. *Generosity* is also an important trait. They are generous with their time, their work, their affection; tending to "forget themselves," even putting at risk their health. And that means displaying a great deal of *energy*, to the point of seeming *tireless.*

Also they think that it is very important to know the history of their communities and their country, and be reminded of them, for that is important to build a strong social identity and for the collective memory from where community members can draw examples, understand attitudes and problems, and find sources of pride. As part of this *historic consciousness*, they also show an *optimistic view of the future*, they trust in the transforming capacity of action and in the possibility to build a better future, working for it in the present. And, therefore, they are *organised* and try to make things in the best way possible, inducing people around them (and doing it themselves) to obtain more *education*, information and specialised *training*. They have a strong *desire for knowledge.*

Finally, they care about social injustice, *reflect* on social contradictions and on socio-economic and political conditions in the country, *rejecting authoritarianism, exclusion and exploitation.* Indeed, these are extraordinary leaders. Very rare to find, but they exist, and luckily, they are part of the contingent of anonymous heroes of everyday life.

AS EXTERNAL AGENTS FOR COMMUNITY CHANGE, WHAT HAVE WE LEARNED?

Leadership then can be a great burden, to which is added anxiety about not having someone to replace them at a certain moment, or to share the tasks. Therefore, in spite of the prestige that community leadership may bring to someone, its costs can also be very high. A solution is distribution of tasks, delegation, and organised participation of other community members, so many people carry out many small tasks. And the sum of all of them, plus leaders' directions and group organisation, allows them to obtain the goals set.

Contact with the two attractive and exasperating kinds of narcissistic-seductive leaders (positive and negative) teaches that the conduct of community action should be in the hands of those with the capacities to carry out the specific tasks needed, and that seduction has its limitations. Therefore a healthy leader rotation should be advisable (that will benefit both stakeholders and leaders), and the largest number of people should participate in the organised groups and in the decisions about activities to be planned and carried out. Also tasks should be subdivided in such a way that the final goal is the outcome of many immediate objectives, guaranteeing thus not only its achievement, but also the participation of many people, their commitment to the community decisions, the distribution of control and direction within the community, avoiding in that way some of the risks of narcissistic leaders.

Critical reflection about actions and their meaning also contributes to avoiding those problems, because through it participants become aware of the fact that community achievements are not the product of a single person. Every effort, both of participants and leaders, should be socially acknowledged and evaluated. No task is so small as not being worthy of attention; no help offered is to be rejected.

REFERENCES

Bass, B. M. (1985). *Leadership and performance beyond expectations.* New York: Free Press.

Domínguez, M. I. (2001). *Informe de pasantía en Psicología Social Comunitaria* [Research assistant report in Community Social Psychology]. Caracas, Venezuela: Universidad Central de Venezuela, Esc. de Psicología.

Farías, L. (2002). *Del bien común como problema íntimo* [Common well-being as an intimate problem]. Caracas, Venezuela: Universidad Central de Venezuela. FACES, Ph.D. Dissertation.

Hernández, E. (1998). Assets and obstacles in community leadership. *Journal of Community Psychology, 26* (3), 261-268.

Montero, M. (1995). *La educación en San José de La Urbina. Dos modelos educativos: Escuela y Biblioteca. Un informe* [Education in San José de La Urbina. Two educational models: School and Library. A report.]. Caracas, Venezuela: Universidad Central de Venezuela, Esc. de Psicología.

Montero, M. (1996). La participación: Significado, alcances y límites [Participation: Meaning, scope and limits]. En Montero, M.; Hernández, E.; Wyssenbach, J.P.; Medina, S., Hurtado, S. & Janssens, A.: *Participación. Ámbitos, retos y perspectivas.* [Participation: Scope, challenges and perspectives]. Caracas, Venezuela: Cesap. Pp. 7-20.

Montero, M. (in press) *New Horizons for Knowledge: The Influence of Citizen Participation.* Chicago, USA: American Psychological Association. Paper presented at the 8th Biennial Conference of the Society for Community Research and Action.

Metadecision:
Training Community Leaders
for Effective Decision-Making

Eneiza Hernández

Organization for Human Experience Development (ODEH), Venezuela

SUMMARY. This article describes an experience in community leadership training, aiming to improve the efficiency of community leaders in their decision-making through metadecision. The concept of metadecision is explained and a training workshop designed and carried out with a group of 42 Venezuelan community leaders in four Venezuelan cities, during the first semester of 2002, is described. The objectives were: (a) to describe the cognition processes behind the decision-making (metadecision) of four groups of community leaders participating in a Community Leaders Training Programme; (b) evaluate the changes produced by that specific training in the decision-making of these community leaders. To measure those changes a questionnaire was used as pretest and posttest. The posttest was applied two months after each workshop in each city. Also, each participant kept a field diary where they would register their observations, impressions and personal findings. Although a quasi-experimental design was used, the data analysis

Address correspondence to: Eneiza Hernández, Universidad Central de Venezuela, Apdo. 80394. Prades del Este, Caracas, 1080-A, Venezuela (E-mail: <eneiza@yahoo.es>).

[Haworth co-indexing entry note]: "Metadecision: Training Community Leaders for Effective Decision-Making." Hernández, Eneiza. Co-published simultaneously in *Journal of Prevention & Intervention in the Community* (The Haworth Press, Inc.) Vol. 27, No. 1, 2004, pp. 53-70; and: *Leadership and Organization for Community Prevention and Intervention in Venezuela* (ed: Maritza Montero) The Haworth Press, Inc., 2004, pp. 53-70. Single or multiple copies of this article are available for a fee from The Haworth Document Delivery Service [1-800-HAWORTH, 9:00 a.m. - 5:00 p.m. (EST). E-mail address: docdelivery@ haworthpress.com].

was qualitative: content answers and field notes were analysed. Results show that the trained leaders had a cognitive reorganisation that enriched their decision-making process. This was expressed in six points: (1) They changed both the tendency to simplify the concept, and their relationship with the decision-making; (2) They valued more the reflection and consultation at the time of decision, assuming a protagonist role in relation to the decision made; (3) They enriched the procedure following the decision-making; changing from a process centred in the decision, to a self- reflective process that facilitated the internal dialogue; (4) They incorporated new information into their decision-making; (5) They became aware of the necessity to handle the complexity in the decisions, and the balance between the dimensions of the process; (6) They were aware of their own self-efficacy and improvement in the efficiency at the moment of decision-making. The participants attributed these changes to the experience lived and acquired during the metadecision training workshop. *[Article copies available for a fee from The Haworth Document Delivery Service: 1-800-HAWORTH. E-mail address: <docdelivery@haworthpress.com> Website: <http://www.HaworthPress.com> © 2004 by The Haworth Press, Inc. All rights reserved.]*

KEYWORDS. Metacognition, metadecision, decision-making, leadership, community development

DECISION-MAKING:
ITS IMPORTANCE AND FACTORS
AFFECTING ITS EFFICIENCY

Decision-making is a process of deliberation, present all along human life, through which people select between possible alternatives in situations where a problem must be solved or some necessity must be satisfied (Ríos, 2000; D'Adamo, 1999; Hernández, 2002). Through decision-making people carry out actions that have effects and produce changes over the world surrounding them. These acts go from the most simple, such as getting up in the morning, for example, to the most complex, such as assuming a specific ethic, political, religious or social standpoint or taking actions that can affect the community.

As an act of election, decision-making has a historic sense. It is produced in a quotidian context that transcends whoever makes the decision. This transcendence resides in the fact that it affects the present and becomes a base for the future, both for the decision-making person, and for those people related to these decisions (Hernández, 2002). This is particularly relevant in the case of community leaders, who often are amidst problematic situations in which they must make complex decisions that imply assuming a position regarding issues or people; to choose between proposals, or act in circumstances that could influence the future of the projects they are leading. For community leaders, effective decision-making is a key factor, one of the more important challenges they must face, since deciding can imply the possibility of defining their actions in the project in which they are taking part, and defining their own place in the world (Ríos, 2000). Nevertheless, efficiency in deciding is affected by factors that frequently are ignored by community leaders.

Some of the more frequent factors are:

1. *Having little awareness of the meaning and importance of the decision-making:* For a decision to be successful, it is necessary that whoever makes it manages sufficient information and has the clearest idea regarding the action being processed and its objectives (Rodríguez, 1988).

   Studies and experiences reported by various researchers and community educators (Burón, 1996; D'Adamo and Calabró, 1998; Martin, 1998) have found that people (especially those in leading places) when making decisions have the tendency to not think about the act of decision. They have no idea of its importance and meaning; they are not clear about what they want to achieve with the decision, and even more, many times they ignore the fact that they are making decisions. In many cases, decisions are made on the base of institutional connections, or are influenced by the information given by closely related people, or simply according to internal states, without taking into account more data (Deshpande, Schoderbek and Joseph, 1994).

2. *Imbalance in the management of emotional, conceptual and instrumental dimensions:* In decision-making are present conceptual, affective and practical elements (Robbins, 1991; Rodríguez, 1998; Puente, 1995). These elements are part of the decision and become characteristic dimensions. Depending on the necessity to be solved, some dimension may be predominant in the decision. This allows for making the following classification (Hernández,

1996): (a) Conceptual decisions, which are characterized by abstractions and logical reasoning; definitions; paradigms: ideological, moral or religious principles; for example, when someone decides which career to study, or when one assumes a position in relation to a given situation or fact; (b) Emotional decisions, which are directed to the satisfaction of some necessity related to emotions such as fear, love, anger or rage, happiness or sadness; for example, when someone decides who is a friend, or when someone decides to express love or anger; and (c) Instrumental decisions, which point to achievement of a concrete effect that satisfies a material necessity or facilitates a task; for example, when someone decides what task they are going to do or which technique they are going to use.

The conceptual, emotional and instrumental dimensions are in constant interaction, and the balance achieved among them will be a determining factor in the decision-making. The dominant dimension in the decision becomes the energizing base and the other two become supportive dimensions. For example, when a community leader decides to conduct a proposal that is to be managed at local or national level, it is more convenient that s(he) assumes it from the perspective of values, principles and paradigms, that is, as a *conceptual* decision. But to be effective it is necessary that the *emotional* dimension be present, such as love for people; sensibility towards related problems; sensibility in relation to other people's emotions. And also the *instrumental* dimension must be present, such as a concrete possibility to implement what is being proposed, consequences for the leader, for the others and for the project. In my experience with community leaders, it is not easy to manage the balance between dimensions, and very seldom they identify the predominant dimension in a proper manner.

3. *Distortions of cognitive representations:* Oftentimes cognitive representations such as beliefs, judgements, values, mental maps, self-image, among others, turn into rigid structures or schemata distorting their reality (Beck, 1979; Robbins, 1991; Colina, 1994; Watzlawick, Beavin and Jackson, 1995; Ríos, 2000; Hernández, 2002). They are learned schemata from previous experiences that can generate emotional or cognitive states driving people to assume dichotomised positions; to generalize opinions; to reduce or to magnify facts and possibilities; to idealize or condemn situations or to omit possible consequences of their acts, independently

of their being positive or negative. These schemata affect the decisions, in the measure that the person ignores key aspects of the situations in which s(he) is deciding and acting according to data that is not corresponding with the real facts.

4. *Difficulty in assuming the consequences of their decisions:* Deciding implies to opt for an alternative. This has consequences and involves a personal responsibility that many times is difficult to assume, and is not transferable. This condition is present in two dilemmas: (a) when one wishes to enjoy the benefit of a variety of options, but must face the fact that to decide implies renouncing one or more options, and (b) when it is necessary to choose between undesirable alternatives, and a decision must absolutely be made. In these cases the person has the tendency to avoid the conflict and can evade the decision-making, transferring to others the responsibility of the decision or falling into depressive or anxious states (Ríos, 2000; Dollard and Miller quoted by Aragón, 2000: 118).

5. *Insecurity facing the lack of control:* It is said that decisions can be taken in three types of scenarios: (a) certainty, (b) partial information, and (c) uncertainty (Ríos, 2000). In each of these scenarios there is always an inevitable degree of doubt (Robbins, 1991), as decisions may depend on others or are the product of unexpected situations, and often enough carry a mixture of successes and failures that are difficult to control. In these cases, each time someone is going to solve a problem or make a decision, the tendency is to use patterns that, as is indicated by Puente (1995, p. 232), are "functional fixations" that lead that person to retake formulas that have worked in the past. Precisely, as these patterns are handy, the person forgets to explore other alternatives that could be simpler and quicker. This implies a sub-utilization of time; an unnecessary waste of resources, and a stereotyped decision-making that frequently is inadequate.

These five factors can be present any time a decision is to be made. They pose a problem when the person is not conscious of the role that these factors can play in his or her decisions. In this manner the factors appear in hidden ways, affecting the efficiency of the decisions made (D'Adamo and Calabró, 1998). Not taking this into account makes the changes and learning very difficult, because when the person faces the failure of his or her decision, s(he) can look for alternatives, for training, or s(he) may adopt the ways that others have used to solve situations, but still manage his or her decision-making from the same perspective, and that perspective is marked by a cognitive absence.

LOOKING FOR AN ALTERNATIVE WAY TO MANAGE THESE FACTORS AND TO ACHIEVE EFFICIENCY IN DECISION-MAKING: METADECISION

This cognitive absence has been identified in different areas of knowledge, particularly in those related to learning and social behavior. In this work we are referring in particular to the settings in which community leaders act. Research carried out from the cognitive perspective has found that people can develop capacities to cover that absence. That phenomenon has been called metacognition and has been described by Flavell (1978); Brown (1978); Burón (1996) and Dorado (1997), as the capacity of supervision and regulation (monitoring) self-learning, in order to be able to detect what failures and potential one has, and to plot the use of the more convenient strategies for each situation.

There are successful training experiences in metacognition to improve learning (metamemory, metareading); to improve communication (metacommunication); to overcome the state of depression or anxiety (cognitive therapy). All of them have shown that the development of metacognitive abilities improves people's performance. It increases their capacity to remember information and to identify the best way to use it; to understand their own communicational processes; to learn to overcome problems that were considered insurmountable; even overcome depression, anxiety or phobias (Vigotsky, 1925; Beck, 1979; Flavell, 1981; Colina, 1994; Watzlawick, Beavin and Jackson, 1995; Burón, 1996; Jans and Lacler, 1997; Poggioli, 1998; Frawley, 1999; Aragón, 2000).

While carrying out the training of community leaders in their decision-making, we arrived at the concept of *metadecision*. Metadecision is a cognitive process, in which the person acts in a self-reflective manner about his/her decision-making. It is based on skills that are not given in an automatic manner, because whoever resorts to metadecision is not just thinking, but is a person reflecting about her/his thinking; a person that acts and is capable of going further, and acts about his/her actions; a person who talks about his/her own talking; deciding about his/her decisions. This self-reflective process allows the person: (a) to be conscious of the processes and facts affecting the person both in a personal level, in relation with the task to be executed, and regarding the decision-making context; (b) to recover previous knowledge related to the decision-making, which helps to identify both the available resources, and also those that need to be incorporated, so as to assume the decision in an effective manner; (c) to incorporate new information, expanding the frame of reference regarding the decision process, and the procedures that will make the decision-making more effective.

Metadecision is supported by three components of the cognitive system conducive to the supervision and control of what occurs during the execution of a task related to complex processes.

Consciousness: Metadecision implies being conscious, in a reflexive manner, of all the processes involved in deciding. In other words, the person becomes aware of: (a) how his/her key cognitive structures (memory, conscience, language), and complex cognitive processes (knowledge, learning, perception, communication, understanding, decision-making, among others) are working, (b) which are the dominant tendencies in her/his cognitive representations or mental models (symbols, schemata, maps, plans, paradigms, beliefs, scripts, strategies, and others) and over all, (c) which factors come into play when s(he) faces the task of deciding.

Knowledge: Metacognitive knowledge is the one developed around the stored experiences of one's own cognitive processes, as well as of the strategic knowledge and the proper use of this knowledge (Flavell, 1993; Hernández, 1998; Paris, Lipson and Wixon, 1983). Metadecision, then, is to know about decision-making and about the matter one is to decide, as well as about the knowledge of the variety of alternatives one counts on, according to the context and the situation in which one must decide. At the same time, it implies that the person knows his or her own characteristics as a subject that makes decisions.

Learning: Metadecision includes the capacity to learn from a metacognitive perspective. This mode of learning implies that the person making decisions is in a permanent process of acquisition of new knowledge that improves her/his abilities and skills, enriching or transforming her/his values and attitudes (Hernández, 1998; Ríos, 2000). This learning process is shown through concrete changes in the mode of deciding, in the incorporation of new means, strategies, procedures or resources, and over all, in the situated use of them.

TRAINING COMMUNITY LEADERS IN METADECISION

Considering that with metadecision it is possible to learn to make effective decisions, a training program was implemented for four groups of community leaders in the Venezuelan cities of Caracas, Maracaibo, Maracay and Valera. The participants were chosen because they had expressed their difficulty in achieving effective decision-making, in spite of having participated in diverse workshops on methods of decision-making.

A training workshop for community leaders was designed in order to develop strategies and foster the construction of personal ways of decision-making. This workshop tackled through exercises the procedure and the contents of the decision-making. The workshop had the following objectives:

1. To describe the cognitive processes underlying the decision-making (metadecision) of the community leaders participating in the Training Program of Community Leaders (TPCL).
2. To evaluate the changes produced in the decision-making process in these community leaders, once they participated in a metadecision training workshop.

Emphasis was put on giving the participants the possibility to have metacognitive experiences, aiming to produce changes in their tendency to make decisions in an automatic way. The development of metadecision skills through the use of five methodological principles and the exploration of three key cognitive processes in decision-making was stressed.

Methodological Principles

Experience as the basis for action: This means having as point of departure for the activities, the person's daily experiences, and deriving from them the basic input to unchain processes of conscientization, while incorporating new knowledge.

Action-Reflection-Action: The specific examples used in the training came from the decision-making practice of the community leaders. They were asked to identify situations, to reflect about them, to elaborate proposals for their transformation, to act again and to evaluate the action. As a basic instrument for use in the workshop, a Manual was used for the participant to describe through exercises and matrixes the processes that s(he) has followed.

Participation: The learning process was effected through individual exercises, readings and group discussion of the processes and concepts, as a way for the community leaders to develop the necessary skills to manage deciding.

Mayeutics: The training facilitator accompanied the process of discovery and conscientization, animating, contributing, posing problems ("problematizing," as Freire said in 1970), challenging, but respecting the leaders' training rhythm.

Group dynamics: Dynamic group techniques were used to stimulate the interaction between the participants (leaders), and propitiate group processes facilitating the raising of consciousness about personal and collective processes implied in the decision-making.

Cognitive Processes

Awareness of decision-making: Community leaders identified the elements they were managing on the following issues: (a) the concept of decision-making, (b) their own way to locate themselves in relation to decision-making, (c) the decision-making procedure they follow, (d) their own strategies to manage balance and the difficulty in decision-making, and (e) their own perception of efficiency.

Revision of existent knowledge: This sub-process goes along with decision-making and implies analysing in depth the five aspects before mentioned.

Learning: The community leaders had the opportunity to incorporate information under three key areas: (a) decision-making, specifically its definition, types, complexity and range, (b) metadecision and metacognition, as well as their influence on the efficiency in decision-making, and (c) mechanisms to make decision-making more effective.

Implementing the Training

Design and validation: The workshop was designed and tested with 20 leaders, to check if the concepts used were clear, and to correct points that could generate confusion. The pilot test was also used to train in decision-making those 20 community leaders, since it would have been unfair to use them as experimental subjects, depriving them of the possibility offered to the other group.

Exploration: Then, the workshop was carried out in each one of the four cities. A questionnaire was applied (pretest) to explore the ways in which the leaders were managing their decision-making, and to describe the process they followed at the time of the decision. The information collected provided a baseline used for the comparison with the data gathered in the posttest.

Intervention: Consisting in the metadecision training workshop for community leaders.

Evaluation: Two months after the intervention, the questionnaire was again applied (posttest) to evaluate the changes produced in the decision-making process and the effects the workshop had on the practice of the participant community leaders.

THE TRAINING WORKSHOP

The workshop was structured in thirteen steps, through which the community leaders executed five activities: (a) an individual exercise: they read the information given to them, and they filled the forms to register their past experiences; (b) they individually analyzed the information and wrote their reflections about it; (c) they shared their reflections with the group; (d) they discussed key aspects the facilitators presented to them; and (e) they wrote their own conclusions on the subjects discussed, pointing out what they had learned.

The Thirteen Steps

Step 1:   Presentation of the workshop, its general frame and the objectives, so the participants would know from the beginning what was expected of them.

Step 2:   Information about decision-making was given to the participants (reading).

Step 3:   Participants' personal diagnosis of their own experience in decision-making.

Step 4:   Identification of the meaning of decision-making based on personal experience (each leader filled a form with the decisions which he or she had made during the past week), and on the information read.

Step 5:   Identification of various forms of decision, using the information read, and an exercise in which the participants located their decisions according to the main dimensions present in the exercise.

Step 6:   Identification of distorted procedures according to information read, and an exercise in which the participants identified the distortions present in their current decisions.

Step 7: Identification of the complexity in decision-making, and personal efficiency according to the information read, and an exercise to classify their decisions according to their complexity.

Step 8: Analysis of the difficulty in a decision due to inefficient management of the emotional, conceptual and instrumental dimensions. The participants filled in a matrix following this recommendation: "Select the decision that has been more difficult for you. Analyze it pointing out: Emotional elements, What inspires me? With what feeling do I relate this situation? Conceptual elements: concepts, values with which I relate the decision. Knowledge of the subject that I have. Information that I handle about the subject. Instrumental elements: What good is it to me? What resources do I have to face it? How is the balance of the dimensions influenced in efficiency or difficulty of the decision?"

Step 9: Analysis of the difficulty. The participants filled a matrix according to the following instructions: "Select a decision that has been difficult or inefficient (could be the same as used in the previous exercise) and analyze it according to the following instructions: In the first column write your goal and the motives that you took into account at the time of the decision. In the second column describe the situation afterwards and explain why it was difficult and inefficient. In the third column describe all the thoughts that came to your mind at the time of the decision; if you do not remember them you can write the thoughts that come to your mind now. In the last line, write the distortions that were (or are) present in the thoughts that work as mediators in the decision."

Step 10: Elaboration of a plan for the transformation of the decision, following this instruction: "Go back to one of the decisions analyzed in the previous exercises and, if you had to make again this decision, decide which aspects you would take into account. What would you drop, what would you add, and what thoughts would accompany the decision?"

Step 11: Metacognitive reflection starting from the person's evaluation of those aspects s(he) was already aware of, and the new aspects that s(he) added to his or her consciousness.

Step 12: Information about metacognition provided by a reading.

Step 13: To close, they were asked to write a brief paragraph on the most important lesson learned in the workshop.

COGNITIVE REORGANIZATION
AS A RESULT OF METADECISION TRAINING

From the analysis and comparison of the answers given in the pre- and posttests by the community leaders, I consider the training as enriching their decision-making process. There was a *cognitive reorganization* shown in both the conception and in the way these leaders related to their decision-making process. This can be proved in six key points:

1. Change in the tendency to simplify the concept and the relation with the decision making, shown in the answers given to the questionnaire items before and after the training had taken place (see Table 1). This change implied an enrichment of the concepts on two levels: The first one related to the defining elements, giving sense to decision making as an action for oneself and for others. This is what is usually communicated regarding the fact being discussed, what it is, and what it is good for (directionality and location). In Table 1, this level is very clear; the decision making has a meaning for the leaders before and after their participation in the training. The second level derives from the previous one and adds elements defining the decision making as a fact in itself, which becomes a *significant*, with its own characteristics. The concept assumes dynamism and becomes a fact that transforms, that can be transformed and that has its own qualities, its implications and its lines of influence. This can be seen in the posttest. Decision making is important when one of the key factors to develop the metadecision process is that the person has a starting point: knowing that decisions are not made in a vacuum, but they are inserted in a history and identity.

2. The participants became aware of the importance of reflection in the transformation of their relationship with the decision-making process, and they assumed more control of the process. This is a key result because reflection and internal dialogue facilitate the access to the information managed by the person about the act s(he) is executing, and this helps her/him to place her/himself in a situated manner in relation to the different alternatives. Besides, that leads the person to become aware of his/her own weaknesses, giving him/her the opportunity to search for efficiency in his/her decisions, assuming control and a protagonist stance (Table 2).

3. As can be seen in Table 3, the participants enriched the procedure for decision making, going from a process centered in the decision

to a self-reflective process. Managing the information in the way described by the community leaders after they received the training facilitates their placing themselves in a situated position. That is important, as it opens the possibility to respond to unexpected changes produced by the circumstances in which the decision is being made. It permits the development of creative ways to decide and act in different situations. In the posttest one finds a person that thinks about him/herself making a decision, someone developing a metadecision process, in the measure that s(he) has given her/himself enough time to become conscious of the processes experienced in the act of deciding.

4. Incorporation and use of new information, as in the case of the notion of balance between conceptual, emotional and instrumental dimensions. Table 4 shows what happened before and after the training. Results of the pretest can be attributed to the fact that the participant did not manage the concept of dimensions and balance between them. But it caught our attention that in the posttest the participants efficiently incorporated the concept from a situated perspective.

5. The participants assumed the necessity to be watchful of the difficulty in the decision making, as can be seen in Table 5. Difficulty is an aspect that goes beyond metadecision skills and is always present. In fact, in the answers given by the community leaders in the pre- and posttest, it is clear that independent of the metacognitive level from which the person relates with the decision making, there is always the need to manage the difficulty. The community leaders participating in this experience said that the most difficult decisions are the emotional ones. That could be explained by the quantity of internal factors implied in that sort of decision.

6. Recognition of both self-efficiency, and the role that the training in metadecision played in the positive transformation of the participants' decision making. In the posttest some questions were included to inquire about the participants' opinions about their efficiency, about the changes in their decision making, and about the influence of the training on these changes. All the participants expressed that they considered themselves more efficient after the training in metadecision, and the explanations they gave for that were related to the workshop as a whole or to specific aspects of it (see Table 6).

TABLE 1. Decision-Making as a Meaning and as a Significant

Decision-making as a meaning		Pretest	Posttest
	What is it?	A process of analysis and selection of alternatives. To act. A capacity.	A process of analysis of causes and consequences of a situation. An important act. To act. To choose between various options. Steps or procedures.
	Objective	To solve problems. To fix goals.	To take position in front of situations. To solve problematic situations. To reach goals.
	Location	In a determined time or situation.	In daily life. In all realms of life.
The decision-making as a significant	Implies	A personal posture. A change.	A personal position. The search for quality.
	Is influenced by		Beliefs Values The environment
	Has influence on		Daily life. On whoever decides. In those people related with whoever decides. The balance with the environment.
	Distinctive Characteristics		The meaning depends on the circumstances. Could be conscious or unconscious. Sometimes it is more effective than others.

TABLE 2. Self-Placing of Community Leaders Facing the Decision-Making

Pretest	Posttest
Almost always they reflect about them	They reflect *always* (daily):
They consider that the control of decisions does not depend on them. They associate the decisions with resignation, personal benefits, uncertainty and obtaining of resources.	They place the control of decisions in themselves. They associate the decisions with motivation, achievement and personal responsibility.
They permanently watch the procedures, causes, indicators, alternatives, results or consequences, and their personal abilities.	They permanently watch: the consequences for them, for others and for the environment. Personal factors apply (values, feelings, efficiency, interests, life project, possibility of assuming consequences). Emotional, conceptual and instrumental balance. Factors associated to the decision itself (implications, options, importance, time, resources, means, reasons).

TABLE 3. Procedure Followed by Community Leaders to Make a Decision

Pretest	Posttest
Decision-making centered in the decision	Decision-making as a self-reflective process
I analyze and make clear the situation or given problem.	I analyze and make clear the situation (visualize the problem, revise if the information is understood, revise resources and supports).
I present and evaluate alternatives.	I consult (search for opinions, revise perspectives, talk with the people implicated, search for external information).
I consult.	I reflect about my position in front of the decision (emotions, feelings, intuitions, ideas).
I analyze the consequences and the feasibility.	I analyze several alternatives (advantages and disadvantages, visualize the scenario).
I plan the strategy.	I reflect over the impact on the environment and on other people.
I make the decision.	I reflect over the benefits that will be obtained (present and future changes).
	I revise the grade of difficulty and the balance between emotional, conceptual and instrumental dimensions.
	I act, I make the decision.

TABLE 4. Management of Conceptual, Emotional and Instrumental Balance

	Pretest	Posttest
Tendency	To be watchful of the balance. *Almost always.*	To be watchful of the balance. *Always.*
Reasons	Varied: to be equilibrate; for the good of all; because it is important; depends on the environment and the situation.	Because the effective and efficient decisions depend on the balance in the dimensions.
Predominance	One dimension tends to be predominant, especially the conceptual ones.	Predominates the tendency to include the three types of decision and to consider the three dimensions in one decision.
Explanations	Always analyze before making a decision. Six participants did not give any explanation.	Search for the balance of the three dimensions. Depends on the moment and the situation.

TABLE 5. Management of Difficulty of the Decisions

	Pretest	Posttest
Tendency	The predominant tendency is to consider it difficult.	The predominant tendency is to consider that it can be: difficult, partially difficult, or simple (whichever of the three).
Origin of difficulty	The social, economic and political impact. Implies a personal responsibility. Takes time and resources. Implies uncertainty.	Depends on the situation (implications, impact on me and others). Depends on the person (on the way to cope with the situation).
Major difficulty	The emotional decisions.	The emotional decisions.
Explanations	Affects in a personal level. Affects others. It is possible to make mistakes.	Involves personal aspects (my emotions, impulses, behavioral patterns). Because it affects people I am involved with.

TABLE 6. Reasons Why the Community Leaders Were More Efficient After the Training

They assumed in an assertive manner decisions that were postponed earlier.
They were open to reflection and changes.
They improved their relationship with the decision-making context.
They obtained the expected results.
They learned to respect their decisions and those of the others.
They searched for balance between dimensions (taking in account others as well as the context).
They planned and evaluated the process of decision-making.
They incorporated the concepts of metadecision and metacognition.
They had developed more personal efficiency about the decision-making process.
They learned to take into account the other people involved when they make decisions.
They developed skills to evaluate the situations in which they make decisions.
They discovered the importance of studying decision-making and looking for the information that permits going deep into it.

CONCLUSION

Community leaders can improve their efficiency in decision making through training in metadecision. As they acquire metacognitive skills that help them to identify the key factors in such processes, they overcome the cognitive absence that often affects decision-making processes. They also became more flexible when standing up to the situations in which they must make a decision.

Metadecision does not impede the person feeling pressure generated by the decision making. What it brings out is the possibility of the person becoming aware of the tools available to her/him and of how they can be used in an adequate manner. It allows making decisions being conscious of the distinctive aspects involved in that act, and doing so in a more efficient way; strengthening their decisions and enriching their information base through the search and incorporation of new data. Two months after the training, the participants said that their major difficulty was related to the emotional aspects, something that in the community work has been detected as a motivating factor, but one that also could be a hurdle for community work (León and Montenegro, 1998). Moreover, emotions of every kind are inevitable, and one of the characteristics of community work is the affective proximity (positive or negative) present in many communities.

Considering that the participatory character of community work makes even more complex the decision-making process, training in metadecision should be recommended as way to deal in a more efficient and conscious way with that important process, not only for those leaders formally recognized as such, but also for those stakeholders in organized groups within the communities.

REFERENCES

Aragón D. J. (2000). *La Psicología del Aprendizaje*. Caracas, Venezuela: San Pablo.

Beck, A.T. (1979). *Cognitive therapy and the emotional disorders*. New York: New American Library.

Burón, J. (1996*). Enseñar a aprender. Introducción a la Metacognición. Recursos e instrumentos psicopedagógicos* (3d. ed.). Madrid, Spain: Mensajero.

Brown, A. (1978). Knowing when, where and how to remember: A problem of metacognition. In R. Glaser (Ed.). *Advances in Instructional Psychology*. Hillsdale, NJ: Erlbaum. Vol. 1.

Colina, L. (1994). *Terapia cognitiva. Cómo manejar la depresión, la ansiedad, los ataques de pánico y las fobias*. Caracas, Venezuela: Gremica.

D'Adamo, O. (1999). Los procesos de toma de decisión in situaciones de conflicto. Percepciones recíprocas y racionalidades implícitas. En *La psicología al fin del siglo* (57-67). Caracas, Venezuela: Sociedad Interamericana de Psicología.

D'Adamo, O. & Calabró, M. (1998). Fases y dinámica de los conflictos. Las racionalidades subyacentes. La guerra de las Malvinas. *Psicología Política, 16*, 7-25.

Deshpande, S., Schoderbek, P. P. & Joseph, J. (1994). Promotion decision by managers: A dependence perspective. *Human Relations, 47* (2), 223-231.

Dorado, C. (1997). Aprender a aprender. Estrategias y técnicas. In *Proyecto Estrateg.* http://pie.xtec.es/cdorado/cdora>/esp./reflexio.Htm.

Flavell, J.H. (1978). Metacognitive development. In J.M. Scandura & C.J. Brainerd (Eds). *Structural/process theories of complex human behaviour.* Rockville, MD: Sijthoff & Noordhoff.

Flavell, J.H. (1981). Cognitive Monitoring. In W.P. Dickson (Ed.) *Children's oral communication skills.* New York: Academic Press.

Flavell, J.H. (1993). *El desarrollo cognitivo.* Madrid, Spain: Aprendizaje Visor.

Frawley, W. (1999). *Vygotsky y la ciencia cognitiva.* Barcelona, Spain: Paidós.

Hernández, E. (1996). *Taller de toma de decisiones.* Caracas, Venezuela: Grupo Social CESAP.

Hernández, E. (2002). *Procesos metacognitivos y toma de decisiones en líderes comunitarios.* Caracas, Venezuela: Universidad Católica Andrés Bello (Dissertation).

Hernández, G. (1998). *Paradigmas en Psicología de la Educación.* México: Paidós.

León, A. & Montenegro, M. (1998) The return of emotion in psychosocial community research. *Journal of Community Psychology, 26* (3), 36-48.

Martín, M. (1998). *Informe del Proyecto de Facilitadores Populares.* Caracas, Venezuela: Grupo Social CESAP.

París, S., Lipson, M. & Wixon, K. (1983). Becoming a strategic reader. Contemporary. *Educational Psychology, 8,* 293-316.

Poggioli, L. (1998). *Estrategias Metacognoscitivas.* Caracas, Venezuela: Fundación Polar.

Puente, A., Poggioli, L. & Navarro, A. (1995). *Psicología Cognoscitiva. Desarrollo y Perspectivas.* Caracas: McGraw Hill.

Ríos, C. P. (2000). *La aventura de aprender.* Caracas, Venezuela: Cognitus.

Robbíns, S. (1991). *Comportamiento organizacional.* México. Prentice-Hall.

Rodríguez, E. M. (1988). *Manejo de problemas y toma de decisiones.* México Manual Moderno.

Vigotsky, L.S. (1925/1997). In *Obras escogidas.* Madrid, Spain: Aprendizaje Visor.

Watzlawick, P., Beavin, J. & Jackson, D. (1995). *Teoría de la comunicación humana.* Barcelona, Spain: Herder.

Community and Families:
Social Organization and Interaction Patterns

Maria Luisa Lodo-Platone

Universidad Central de Venezuela

SUMMARY. The purpose of this paper is to present the social organization, social networks and interactive processes supporting family systems living in communities with marginal economies, in disadvantaged neighbourhoods (barrios) in Caracas, Venezuela. Twelve families inserted in four different communities were observed by four researchers, taking thirty-six ethnographic records of the families' daily life activities, as well as the interaction patterns between family members, and between the family system and the community and social organizations. Some characteristics of the organization, structure, and functioning of the underprivileged family systems as well as their interrelations to the community and to the educational and social institutions are shown. It is concluded that the analysis of these interactive patterns permits the researcher to explore the complexity of family life in poverty stricken communities, its culture and process of change. *[Article copies available for a fee from The Haworth Document Delivery Service: 1-800-HAWORTH.*

Address correspondence to: Maria Luisa Lodo-Platone, Universidad Central de Venezuela, Instituto de Psicología Apartado Postal 47363, Caracas, 1041-A, Venezuela (E-mail: mplatone@reacciun.ve).

This paper was written at the Center for Educational Research (TEBAS), at Universidad Central de Venezuela, as part of The Community Ethnographic Observations Project.

[Haworth co-indexing entry note]: "Community and Families: Social Organization and Interaction Patterns." Lodo-Platone, Maria Luisa. Co-published simultaneously in *Journal of Prevention & Intervention in the Community* (The Haworth Press, Inc.) Vol. 27, No. 1, 2004, pp. 71-87; and: *Leadership and Organization for Community Prevention and Intervention in Venezuela* (ed: Maritza Montero) The Haworth Press, Inc., 2004, pp. 71-87. Single or multiple copies of this article are available for a fee from The Haworth Document Delivery Service [1-800-HAWORTH, 9:00 a.m. - 5:00 p.m. (EST). E-mail address: docdelivery@haworthpress.com].

http://www.haworthpress.com/web/JPIC
Digital Object Identifier: 10.1300/J005v27n01_06

*E-mail address: <docdelivery@haworthpress.com> Website: <http://www.
HaworthPress.com>* © 2004 by The Haworth Press, Inc. All rights reserved.]

KEYWORDS. Family system, underprivileged communities, social organization, interactive processes

This paper presents an analysis of family systems interactions and networks promoting both the consolidation of family ties, and the bonds these families have with their community (Bronfenbrenner, 1977, 1979). The importance of this study has to do with the need to develop a theoretical understanding of contemporary underprivileged family systems and their relations with the communities they belong to. These systems deal with people's everyday activities and concerns, the relationship between public and private activities, and the structural and adaptive changes that may happen within their communities.

In the first section of the paper the theoretical references and the methodological framework of the study are discussed, and a description is given of the data sources and procedures used in data collection and processing. A second section describes the results in order to provide an understanding of the social environment of the family systems. This section begins by describing the four communities studied. Several topics are discussed concerning family structure and functioning, as well as family interactions with the school and the community systems. Finally, a summary of the main findings is presented in the conclusions.

THEORETICAL FRAMEWORK

Nowadays, there is considerable reflection going on concerning emergent research paradigms. These are usually presented in opposition to the positivist perspective that is considered to be deficient in relation to the promotion of social change (Platone, 1983, 1998). It is supposed that this change can only be understood in relation to varied and integrated theoretical formulations that contain linguistic, philosophical, ecological, holistic and humanistic aspects.

This integration has epistemological connotations. Because of the complexity of the factors that must be taken into account, it has become necessary to find comprehensive conditions for the management of symbols and meanings in a coherent way, since meaning is related to historical and cultural interpretations. In this paper, "culture" has to do with specific ways of feeling, thinking, and acting which are expressed in discourse and used to clarify people's identities. Differences in these areas also point to social differences between people in the same community.

Derrida (1991) suggests that our everyday experience takes form within the cultural framework of collective discourse. We cannot free ourselves from the ideological structure in which we live. Discourse is a cultural creation that allows social norms to be transmitted. These norms are tightly related to the power relations of the groups in which the discourse occurs. Collective discourse is affected by cultural traditions; it is supported by political structures and is institutionalized through everyday practices. Everyday reality is constructed through language. Meaning is assigned to face-to-face social interaction in which people are aware of sharing experiences. The inter-subjective and cultural aspects of living coincide, appearing then as the content of everyday conversations (Derrida, 1974; Fernández-Christlieb, 1994; Gergen, 1991; Shotter, 1993).

Everyday life is considered here to be a space in which social relations are systematic and organized through direct action and communication. The established social order is expressed and reproduced in the context of daily life. For this reason, commonplace existence can be both authentic, alienated, and detached from the rest of society (Esté, 1995). Montero (1987, 1991) states that everyday life is the area of experience that most easily becomes alienated, because it is so encumbered with values and ideological meaning.

On the other hand, interaction is the interpersonal process for the social construction of reality. A phenomenological analysis of interaction begins with the meaning of communication that occurs in a social context. This research is theoretically oriented by a constructionist-interactionist framework. It adopts a system and structural perspective that considers reality to exist in the sense that people actually "live" and perceive it. Emphasis is given both to the events that have significance for people and to the natural context of the functional ecosystem in which they occur.

METHODOLOGICAL FRAMEWORK

There is not much information in the literature about the cultural, communicational and social organization of Venezuelan underprivileged families. For this reason in this paper an ethnographic approach was employed. The *III National Neighborhood Register* (Fundacomún and OCEI, 1993) was used to locate 32 barrios representing 8% of the universe of all the barrios in Caracas. From these, four barrios were intentionally selected. They are located approximately at the metropolitan area's four compass points, and include: (1) Las Minitas (East), (2) Raúl Leoni II (West), (3) Blandín (North), and (4) Las Torres (South). The information given in the Register was complemented with knowledge provided by the people interviewed and community observation.

Strategies Used in Data Collection

Data collection instruments were developed in a process of successive adaptations made by the field workers assigned to the work. The final instruments were the following:

a. An ethnographic description of community social areas in which the inhabitants of the barrios tend to get together (meeting places).
b. Interviews with barrio residents.
c. An ethnographic general description of the barrio family.
d. An ethnographic description of the families studied.
e. Family narratives.

In this study we define *ethnographic description* as a set of descriptions carried out by a researcher who keeps field notes about social processes observed in the families' homes and in other places used for social encounters. Each researcher (four in total) described three families. That included three observations obtained by each researcher for different instances of social interaction in each place described.

Interview Procedures

Two open-ended interviews of one hour each were carried out regarding the lives of the persons interviewed. The final product of these conversations was termed "biographical narratives" (Marinas, 1990). They are shorter than "life histories" and do not go into as much detail. However, the interviewer encouraged the interviewees to spend time discussing a particular point when they desired to do so. The interviews can be described in the following way:

They were open conversations about family history and their relationship with community affairs. Especially important were family origins and growth, religious beliefs, other beliefs, political participation, and frequent activities.

The texts were interpreted, both in terms of the content and certain formal aspects such as reiterations and omissions. Attention was paid to the relation between microsocial and macrosocial distinctions (Guitián, 1993). This method allows the researchers to relate economic, political, religious, community and social aspects of the lives of the interviewees with other experiences they describe. Thus, many different areas of experience can be described subjectively and can be linked to social organization and functioning.

THE BARRIOS AS CONTEXT FOR COMMUNITIES

The "Blandín" barrio was founded in 1920 and has a population of 6,342 people, which is considered as high density in proportion to its geographical area. "Las Minitas" (Little Mines) started in 1967 and has actually a population of 2,830. The community "Las Siete Hermanas" (The Seven Sisters) was founded in 1993; "Raúl Leoni II" (a president's name) in 1984. Neither of these two was surveyed by the Register mentioned above so the population ciphers are unknown.

These four communities were approached simultaneously. Access was achieved in one of two ways. Either a member of the research team was introduced to community members by someone from the local parish, or team members began to frequent plazas, shops, bars or workshops where people tended to gather, in order to identify community leaders. Later the researchers would tour the barrio walkways, stairways (in the uphill communities), and alleys. In these excursions the researchers would chat with people, and take notes on the community history and structure.

Most of the people belonging to these communities had originally migrated from agrarian regions of Venezuela to Caracas. At that time they were anticipating a better standard of living. Some families, however, were immigrants from other countries, mainly from Colombia, who were drawn to Venezuela by the oil price boom in the seventies.

Most were squatters. Some had gradually occupied the land on which their houses were built, but others did it abruptly. In every case the municipal authorities considered squatting illegal. The National Guard engaged in impossible "resistance struggles" against those who began clandestine constructions. Said one resident: "When they demolished them in the daytime, we would rebuild them by night." When one member of an extended family managed to get his shanty built, he let his relatives know, so they would come and put up their own shanties beside the original one, or enlarge it. They would put up small contiguous units in which relatives could be close together, sharing child-care responsibilities and resources. The family organization is "matrifocal" because the mother, aunt or grandmother is the affective and organizational center of the family (Recagno, 1998).

First residents tend to reject newcomers. Their higher status resides in their houses being located nearer to the access road or on the equivalent of a Main Street. Also, because having arrived earlier, they have had time to obtain funds to have their houses better kept and make them more solid. Often they keep pets and other domestic animals such as chickens, and they plant fruit trees or vegetables when they have enough space to do so. Initially, the shanties are built of inexpensive materials, and sometimes of scavenged materials such as wooden boards, zinc foil, cardboard, and cinder blocks. As the family feels sure about staying in those places, the dwelling is little by little transformed, building materials become more resistant, and doors, cement floors and other details are added.

Often the constructions lack public services such as fresh water, plumbing, and garbage collection. Because of this, the presence of flies, mosquitoes, and vermin increase health problems. Children can frequently be seen playing in dirty water. Also, because of the precarious nature of the constructions, landslides are a continual danger in the rainy season. To obtain electricity, the residents climb the poles that sustain the municipal wires and illegally "tap" into them. Transportation is available up to the places that jeeps or double-traction station wagons can reach. It also is expensive and hard to obtain, and people have to form long lines at rush hours to get to school or work.

In general, the barrio can be considered as an ecosystem for the families that live there. It is the stage on which the family and the social group interact and where everyday activities take place.

FAMILY INTERACTION:
ORGANIZATION, STRUCTURE AND FAMILY FUNCTIONING

A systemic stance is used here to refer to family and community interaction. Families are considered as complex and open systems that undergo continuous transformations. They are located within a context that we call an *ecosystem* (Bateson, 1960-1970; von Bertalanffy, 1950; Buckley, 1967).

The family system is made up of the families' behavioral sequences, their interactions, and the communications that occur between the family members. Observation of these elements permits the researcher to infer the family organization, structure, and functioning. In a similar sense, an analysis of the meanings and symbols generated at the community level can help clarify family structures.

In what follows, the results of ethnographic observations and text analysis of family conversations will be discussed. The observations were made in community and home settings. The analysis was structured in terms of the relational and functional dynamics of family organization and structure.

Family Structure

By the triangulation of the 36 ethnographic records collected and the open interviews of the twelve families, it was found that in the family structure of the four barrios there is a prevalence of unstable relationships in the conjugal subsystem as a consequence of extreme poverty.

On the other hand, the family structure is centered on the mother figure, who is the responsible adult around which the household and children are united. She also represents the affective and organizational center of the family system. The mother-figure tends to be mythified, in contrast to the father-figure, who is considered peripheral.

Younger children are often left to be taken care of by older siblings. It is frequent for the grandmother, aunt or godmother to take over the responsibility of the children when the mother has to work. Along with the mother, they form the executive and affective centers of the family. Thus the extended family is an important support for raising children.

In the barrios, it is common to find "a modified extended family network" of kinfolk sharing a common space, where different adjacent units are added to the structure of the house when grown-up children get married. This network is also an important resource for looking after children and giving families support. On some occasions, children are left alone in the house or in the streets, under the occasional surveillance of a collaborative neighbour. Thus friends and neighbors in the community also provide important social support for the family.

Families suffer economic difficulties and their needs cannot be sufficiently provided for because of the costs involved in supporting many children. Those from the mother's previous unions usually live with her. Fathers contribute to the support of their children within their current unions, but usually do not contribute much to children from their previous unions, usually living in other households. Thus, mothers usually bear the main burden in the economic support of the household.

The time span during which children are protected from work is very short. Ten-year-old children are already expected to report some benefits to the family, such as doing chores in the house, picking up bottles and cans to sell, carrying water to the house, helping peddle products made by the mother (e.g., pastries or sweets) and so on.

Family Functioning

Five aspects of family organization were taken into account: (a) daily problem solving, (b) family communication, (c) behavioral patterns in the designation of responsibilities within the household, (d) authority, supervision and control standards, and (e) affective relationships and the reciprocal expressions of feelings. These dimensions are proposed by Epstein, Bishop and Levin (1978), and Platone (1983).

a. Daily problem solving

In daily life, there is little planning to avoid possible problems. Though lack of money makes it difficult to provide for the morrow, people often express the fatalistic idea that there is no use in anticipating problems; they are to be confronted when they present themselves. Thus, solutions are usually improvised on the spur of the moment. Often such solutions have negative effects on other areas of life.

b. Communication patterns

Communication among family members usually refers to the events of the day. Often it is reduced because members prefer to watch TV. Communication about shared problems is often avoided because of the disagreeable effects of inadequate communication patterns.

c. Behavioral patterns

There are few routine behavioral patterns related to the designation of responsibilities within the household. When it is necessary to maintain the stability of the family system, members show great flexibility in performing different roles and functions, especially those related to child rearing and protection.

d. Authority, supervision and control standards

The mother tends to be the authority figure of the household. However, there is little consistency in setting norms or disciplining the children, mainly because the mother is at work during the day. For this reason, any adult or older sibling may exercise the supervision and control of the younger children. Physical punishments are more frequent than other disciplinary methods. The communication of norms and expectations about appropriate behavior tends to be vague and inexplicit.

e. Affective relationships and the reciprocal expression of feelings

Families defend their members from outsiders and consider loyalty to each other very important. Members rally around when someone is in difficulties.

From these observations, other conclusions emerge. The families have enormous vitality and capacities for adapting to adverse circumstances. Strong affective and loyalty bonds are established between the family core and the extended family, and affective bonds and cooperation are also established among neighbors. In this way natural networks for providing mutual support are generated, creating a web within the community. The family members are also very flexible to perform different roles to maintain the stability of the system, especially in relation to child rearing and protection.

THE PARTICIPATION OF FAMILY SYSTEMS IN ORGANIZED COMMUNITY LIFE

The interaction patterns that the members of the disadvantaged family systems establish with the community of the barrios were observed through their participation in both informal gatherings and political meetings for discussing collective problems. In all four barrios studied, it was found that community life is organized in terms of family and social networks of neighbors.

Conversation topics turn around meaning attributed to their everyday life and to the community through the experience of events occurring in a common space and time. In this way they also construct a common history and consolidate their emotional ties as members of the community. Shared history, symbols, and common stories are central to the process of community organization and the maintenance of community boundaries. As Nagel (1994: 163) states, "culture is constructed in much the same way as ethnic boundaries are built, by the action of indi-

viduals and groups and their interaction with the larger society."
Through these interaction processes community life is consolidated and
emotional ties are established. And thus, the history, experiences, emotions and symbols that members of human systems share provide the
foundations for developing a sense of community.

On the other hand, these informal gatherings and conversations lead
to a critical analysis of the events and community circumstances (e.g.,
delinquent members, drug dealings, inequalities and insufficiency, as
well as needs and strengths). As found in the analysis of some conversations, they also contribute to building up community cohesion, solidarity, and a sense of belonging. So, for example, the people interviewed
said: " . . . this is my barrio"; "here I know everybody and receive support when I need it."

Assemblies and other meetings take place wherever all the people
can fit together. That is, in school buildings, plazas, garages, or even
people's homes. Convocation is made by word-of-mouth, and that
means that people who live far from the center of the barrio may not
hear about them. Attendance depends on what is to be discussed. Two
typical discussion topics are described here:

1. A building made for community purposes by the government was
   later abandoned. The community met to decide what to do with it.
   One person wanted to transform it into a cultural meeting place.
   This person felt that the "Neighbors' Association," a type of community organization legally recognized, should handle things.

2. A basketball space was considered inadequate by some community
   members. One community member complained saying: "There's a
   ring, but it doesn't even have a basket on it." Another one said:

   > In the rainy season it looks like a swimming pool and the kids
   > kick water at each other, slide on the slippery surfaces, and ride
   > bikes in the mud. It's even been used as a dance floor, a chil-
   > dren's park, a place for couples to meet, and other activities that
   > are not all that healthy.

In such meetings, community members express their intentions of
participating in activities for community improvement.

These examples reveal how individuals form a pattern of shared attitudes, beliefs, norms and values that is organized around a subject that

is meaningful to the people of the community, spoken in a particular common language. These conversations conform to patterns of organization related to the community and their environment to draw on different sources to work together to solve problems for the collective well-being.

However, the fragility of the community's conditions makes it difficult to produce a cohesive community action. The lack of public services, communication means, financial resources, as well as the serious health, educational and work situations affecting the family and the organized groups of the community, are obstacles for a community cohesive self-organization. There is the need for an alternative political action to support and consolidate the community members' efforts, especially when the social context is under drastic political and socioeconomic changes, as is currently happening in Venezuela.

As Montero (1998; 76) suggests, this action should be organized "following horizontal and circular models . . . which enable a greater number of people to have access to the decision-making processes and participation with greater commitment." Also, it is necessary: (a) to empower the community family systems in capabilities and resources through workshops for specific problems; (b) to reinforce the actual supporting networks and to establish new ones; and (c) to provide alternative ways of actions to consolidate families as members of the community.

FAMILY AND SCHOOL SYSTEM INTERACTION

The people interviewed usually described the schools as places in which personal contact is evaded, and as unconnected with the community's daily life. Most frequently, contact between the school and the neighborhood families happened only when parents were summoned by teachers to discuss some child's misbehavior. The PTA meetings can be described as teachers' scoldings that produce mutual distrust. This distrust has its origin in the school personnel's prejudices in relation to the barrio population, a situation coming from the inconsistency between school activities and the community way of life. And that derives from the official programming which is based on the cultural values of an industrial society, which are different from the cultural codes and symbols of the community where the children live (Esté, 1994, 1995, 1996).

Among the effects of the above mentioned discrepancy is a high desertion rate for the schools (approximately 42% from first through sixth grade). Sometimes a child is taken out of school because he cannot adapt to the school system. This kind of desertion is related to socioeconomic scarcity; however, there is a high rate of educational exclusion which is mostly due to failure of the school to attend to the peculiar needs of the barrio's families.

Another effect is that the communities do not support the schools. Families consider the schools as government outposts that have nothing to do with their culture and expectations, even though they recognize the importance of education to get a job and to be inserted in the larger society. Furthermore, the contrast between school and community contexts is not motivating for the children for their dissimilar characteristics.

The school system is a bureaucratic structure in which power relations are institutionalized. Families, as we have before discussed, have diffuse, inconsistent and interchangeable power structures. The school has values, beliefs and interaction styles that are different from the families' and the barrio's. For this reason the child's interaction abilities at school and his or her behavior are very different from those he or she develops at home or in the community. On the other hand, both the families and the school belong to a historical tradition that has produced different myths and beliefs.

Some problems that children have in getting to school have to do with the structural conditions of the barrios. For example, public transportation and the availability of fresh water are insufficient. Another problem is political, as the Ministry of Education requires children to have a birth certificate and other legal documents, and some children do not have them because of the family migration, or because illegitimate sons and daughters may have never been "presented" by their parents to the authorities to be registered.

FAMILY AND COMMUNITY ORGANIZATIONS' INTERACTIONS

Poverty marks the lives of families living in marginal economies. They have much interaction with many outside groups, institutions and organizations, but they remain distant from them. The police, welfare groups, and those that distribute food, for example, have the power to make long-lasting decisions for the lives of these people, who often do not understand those institutions' functions, operations, and responsibilities. Even worse, they are ignorant of their own rights and of the ways they might gain entrance to other systems from which they are normally excluded.

The disadvantaged communities are organized in terms of family and social networks. They relate to society in general as though it were a vaguely defined and dangerous monolith. The people in those communities do not understand the linguistic codes, values or criteria of this society from which they are excluded, but they attribute power and prestige to it. The "ones in charge" and the "well-to-do" make up a distant but attractive world enhanced by the mass communication networks, a world that is unattainable for inhabitants of the barrio. Interactive patterns that are reiterative and undifferentiated are formed, not allowing the families to make consistent demands on the environment. Most welfare organizations aiding underprivileged families are influenced by values that are foreign to these people. Medical services, social agencies, and schools support the idea of a traditional, nuclear family, although the families they assist do not have that structure. They label other family structures as deficient and pathological. Then, contact between them and the aid-systems becomes stereotyped and prejudiced. These institutions sometimes use their role as promoter of family welfare to probe the families' everyday activities. This invasion functions as a constraint on family privacy.

As before mentioned, the family structure of these communities is centered on the mother figure, who is the only responsible adult around which the household and children are united. Mothers make up the main communication channel for the family and the social organizations. They are given all the responsibility for the household. This situation produces a vicious circle between the aid-systems and the family system.

The ambiguous cultural conception of women is responsible for "determining" that these families have inherent flaws, in spite of this matrilineal and mother-centered structure being the rule in the country (Vethencourt, 1974; Montero, 1984; Moreno, 1995; Hurtado, 1995a, 1995b; Recagno, 1998). Often women who have the role of head of the family live with their mothers. These women (both mother and grandmother) embody the nuclear family's executive subsystem. It is necessary, therefore, that this role be recognized by schools and social institutions.

RELIGIOUSNESS, SPIRITUALITY AND COMMUNITY INTERACTION

In this paper the word "religiousness" refers to the rituals that form part of people's everyday life. The symbols stream spontaneously from their beliefs rather than from formal doctrines. Religious experience is an interactive process that implies participation in the church rituals as well as the people's interpretation of their own experiences. "Spirituality" is understood here as a searching for meaning related to a "supreme being." It is a world view that forms part of people's everyday lives, but not necessarily participation in an organized religion. In the four barrios we found several organized belief systems that bring families together: the Catholic, the Evangelical, the Pentecostal, and the Jehovah's Witnesses.

The main religion in the country is Catholicism. Every barrio has an easy-to-reach parochial church. Believers attend it on the days of the week when rites are celebrated, and on special occasions, such as religious festivities, marriages, baptisms and first communions. The church also functions as a formal meeting place. Activities that are important for maintaining community cohesion such as young people's meetings and club meetings are held there. Furthermore, certain street events are coordinated by the church, such as processions and community assemblies.

Sometimes a family will have symbols from different denominations, including images associated with the rites and myths of Afro-Latin and spiritist practices (called *Santería*), which was brought by African slaves to Venezuela. Some sort of generalized syncretism in religiosity uniting all the belief systems mentioned above can also be found in the communities we worked with. For example, Mrs. Rosa, a lady living in one of the barrios, is a "santera" consultant whose clients visit her at home. There she gives advice about love, economy, and health problems. Besides making a living, because of that capacity she is a well-known member of the community and performs a sort of leadership. Religiosity and spirituality have functional characteristics for barrio families. They are used at critical moments in family life and as elements that protect the home.

CONCLUSIONS

The more frequent patterns in family functioning were: (a) problems solved on the spur of the moment with little advance planning and a fatalistic "time will solve everything" attitude; (b) infrequent communication between family members about shared problems; (c) flexibility of family members in performing different roles and functions, especially those related to child rearing and protection; (d) though the mother tends to be the authority figure in the household, she is usually at work all day and other available adults supervise and control the children. Thus, there is little consistency in setting norms or disciplining the children. Physical punishments are the usual disciplinary method. Norms and expectations about appropriate behavior tend to be vague and inexplicit; (e) Families defend their members from outsiders and support those in difficulties. Three different types of family structure are to be found: those centered on the mother, those centered on the extended family, and those centered on a modified extended family network of kinfolk. That type of structure constitutes the substratum of community organization. These types and patterns imply an enormous vitality and capacity to adapt to adverse circumstances; flexibility of role taking, especially in relation to child rearing; strong bonds of affection and loyalty are established with members of the family and extended family, as well as with neighbors. Therefore, they generate natural networks to provide mutual support and co-operation.

In their discourse, members of the community express the need to participate in improving community conditions and to solve common problems through organized community associations. The way to do that is through extended families-neighbours networks. Participation in religious festivities and events also helps establish cohesive ties among community residents. Women frequently are heads of families, as well as heads of community-organized groups in charge of problem solving and decision making. It is necessary then that this role be recognized by external agents, especially in the interactions between families and schools, often tense and difficult.

Further research about the relation between family and community organization is needed as families adapt to contexts differently. To strengthen the organization of the social structure of the barrios, it is our understanding that the investigation of family functioning and organization must take into account both everyday dynamics and interrelatedness to social contexts. This will provide a better comprehension of the multiple dimensions emerging from the people's discourse when we consider intervention to promote changes in the family systems and their communities.

REFERENCES

Almedo, G. (1998). *Rastros Escolares en la comunidad.* Caracas, Venezuela: Paper at the VI Meeting of the Humanities and Education Research. Universidad Central de Venezuela.

Bateson, G. (1972). *Steps to an Ecology of Mind.* New York: Chandler Publishing.

Bertalanffy, L. von (1950). An Outline of General Systems Theory. *British Journal of Philosophical Science, 1,* 134:165.

Bronfenbrenner, U. (1977). The changing American Family. In M. Hetherington & Ross D. Parke (Eds.). *Contemporary Reading in Child Psychology*. New York: McGraw-Hill.

Bronfenbrenner, U. (1979). *The Ecology of Human Development*. Boston: Harvard University Press.

Buckley, W. (1967). *Sociology and Modern Systems Theory*. Englewood Cliffs, NJ: Prentice Hall.

Derrida, J. (1991). *A Derrida Reader: Between the Blinds*. New York: Columbia University Press.

Epstein, N.B., Bishop, D.S., & Levin, S. (1978). The McMaster Model of family functioning. *Journal of Marital and Family Therapy, 9,* 171:180.

Esté, A. (1994). *El Aula Punitiva*. Caracas, Venezuela: Tropykos-Tebas.

Esté, A. (1995). *Educación para la dignidad*. Caracas; Venezuela: Tropykos.

Esté, A. (1996). *Migrantes y Excluídos*. Caracas, Venezuela: Ediciones Astro Data.

Fernández-Christlieb, P. (1994). La lógica epistémica de la invención de la realidad. In M. Montero (Ed.), *Conocimiento, realidad e ideología. Fascículo de AVEPSO, 6,* 19-35.

Fundacomún & OCEI (1993). *Indicadores sociodemográficos*. Caracas, Venezuela.

Gergen, K. (1991). *The saturated self: Dilemma of identity in contemporary life*. New York: Basic Books.

Guitián, C. (1993). Familia Popular Urbana: Reconstrucción de un proyecto. *Urbana 12,* 43-56.

Hurtado, S. (1995a). *Cultura Matrisocial y Sociedad Popular en América Latina*. Caracas, Venezuela: Editorial Tropykos-FACES/UCV.

Hurtado, S. (1995b). *Trabajo femenino, fecundidad y familia popular urbana*. Caracas, Venezuela: Universidad Central de Venezuela-CDCH.

Lodo-Platone, M.L. (1997). La familia Venezolana en el discurso de las Ciencias Sociales. *Revista AVEPSO, XX* (2), 59-72.

Marcano, J. (1998). *Sitios de encuentro en las comunidades populares*. Paper at the VI Meeting of the Humanities and Education Research, Caracas, Venezuela: Universidad Central de Venezuela.

Marinas, J.M. (1990). *La historia oral, método y experiencia*. Madrid, Spain: Editorial Debate.

Martínez, M. (1994). *Comportamiento Humano*. México: Trillas.

Mata, M. (1998). *Religiosidad Popular*. Paper given at the VI Meeting of the Humanities and Educational Research, Universidad Central de Venezuela, Caracas.

Montero, M. (1987). *Ideología, alienación e identidad nacional*. Caracas, Venezuela: EBUC.

Montero, M. (1994). Consciousness-raising, conversion and de-ideologization in community psychosocial work. *Journal of Community Psychology, 22* (1) 3-11.

Montero, M. (1998). Psychosocial community work as an alternative mode of political action (The construction and critical transformation of society). *Community, Work & Family, 1* (1) 65-78.

Moreno Olmedo, A. (1995). *La familia Popular Venezolana*. Caracas, Venezuela: Centro Gumilla.

Nagel, J. (1994). Constructing ethnicity: Creating and recreating ethnic, identity and culture. *Social Problems, 41*, 152-176.

Platone, M.L. (1983). *A systems oriented test to measure adaptation patterns of Hispanic elementary school children.* University of Massachusetts at Amherst, Ph.D. Dissertation. University Microfilm International, Michigan DAO 56766. Unpublished.

Platone, M.L. (1998a). Community and Family in Venezuela. Reflections on Paradigms and Theoretical Models. *Community, Work & Family, 1(2)*, 167:178.

Platone, M.L. (1998b). *Conflicto y Violencia en la Familia.* Caracas, Venezuela: Paper at the VI Meeting of the Humanities and Educational Research. Universidad Central de Venezuela.

Recagno, I. (1998). Familia y Exclusión Social. In M.L. Platone (Ed.) *Familia: Trama, Escenario y Drama de los Barrios Populares. Fascículo AVEPSO, 9,* 41-59.

Ruíz, A. (1998). *Legalidad y legitimidad en el barrio.* Paper given at the VI Metting of the Humanities and Educational Research, Universidad Central de Venezuela, Caracas.

Shotter, J. (1993). *Conversational Realities: Constructing Life Through Language.* London: Sage.

TEBAS, Centro de Investigaciones Educativas. (1994-1998). *Registro Etnográfico de Comunidades.* Caracas, Venezuela: Database VIEW 21.

Vethencourt, J. (1974). *La estructura atípica y el fracaso cultural de Venezuela.* Caracas, Venezuela: Centro de Investigaciones Populares.

Career Stress in Changing Times, edited by James Campbell Quick, PhD, MBA, Robert E. Hess, PhD, Jared Hermalin, PhD, and Jonathan D. Quick, MD* (Vol. 8, No. 1, 1990). *"A well-organized book. . . . It deals with planning a career and career changes and the stresses involved." (American Association of Psychiatric Administrators)*

Prevention in Community Mental Health Centers, edited by Robert E. Hess, PhD, and John Morgan, PhD* (Vol. 7, No. 2, 1990). *"A fascinating bird's-eye view of six significant programs of preventive care which have survived the rise and fall of preventive psychiatry in the U.S." (British Journal of Psychiatry)*

Protecting the Children: Strategies for Optimizing Emotional and Behavioral Development, edited by Raymond P. Lorion, PhD* (Vol. 7, No. 1, 1990). *"This is a masterfully conceptualized and edited volume presenting theory-driven, empirically based, developmentally oriented prevention." (Michael C. Roberts, PhD, Professor of Psychology, The University of Alabama)*

The National Mental Health Association: Eighty Years of Involvement in the Field of Prevention, edited by Robert E. Hess, PhD, and Jean DeLeon, PhD* (Vol. 6, No. 2, 1989). *"As a family life educator interested in both the history of the field, current efforts, and especially the evaluation of programs, I find this book quite interesting. I enjoyed reviewing it and believe that I will return to it many times. It is also a book I will recommend to students." (Family Relations)*

A Guide to Conducting Prevention Research in the Community: First Steps, by James G. Kelly, PhD, Nancy Dassoff, PhD, Ira Levin, PhD, Janice Schreckengost, MA, AB, Stephen P. Stelzner, PhD, and B. Eileen Altman, PhD* (Vol. 6, No. 1, 1989). *"An invaluable compendium for the prevention practitioner, as well as the researcher, laying out the essentials for developing effective prevention programs in the community. . . . This is a book which should be in the prevention practitioner's library, to read, re-read, and ponder." (The Community Psychologist)*

Prevention: Toward a Multidisciplinary Approach, edited by Leonard A. Jason, PhD, Robert D. Felner, PhD, John N. Moritsugu, PhD, and Robert E. Hess, PhD* (Vol. 5, No. 2, 1987). *"Will not only be of intellectual value to the professional but also to students in courses aimed at presenting a refreshingly comprehensive picture of the conceptual and practical relationships between community and prevention." (Seymour B. Sarason, Associate Professor of Psychology, Yale University)*

Prevention and Health: Directions for Policy and Practice, edited by Alfred H. Katz, PhD, Jared A. Hermalin, PhD, and Robert E. Hess, PhD* (Vol. 5, No. 1, 1987). *Read about the most current efforts being undertaken to promote better health.*

The Ecology of Prevention: Illustrating Mental Health Consultation, edited by James G. Kelly, PhD, and Robert E. Hess, PhD* (Vol. 4, No. 3/4, 1987). *"Will provide the consultant with a very useful framework and the student with an appreciation for the time and commitment necessary to bring about lasting changes of a preventive nature." (The Community Psychologist)*

Beyond the Individual: Environmental Approaches and Prevention, edited by Abraham Wandersman, PhD, and Robert E. Hess, PhD* (Vol. 4, No. 1/2, 1985). *"This excellent book has immediate appeal for those involved with environmental psychology . . . likely to be of great interest to those working in the areas of community psychology, planning, and design." (Australian Journal of Psychology)*

Prevention: The Michigan Experience, edited by Betty Tableman, MPA, and Robert E. Hess, PhD* (Vol. 3, No. 4, 1985). *An in-depth look at one state's outstanding prevention programs.*

Studies in Empowerment: Steps Toward Understanding and Action, edited by Julian Rappaport, Carolyn Swift, and Robert E. Hess, PhD* (Vol. 3, No. 2/3, 1984). *"Provides diverse applications of the empowerment model to the promotion of mental health and the prevention of mental illness." (Prevention Forum Newsline)*

Aging and Prevention: New Approaches for Preventing Health and Mental Health Problems in Older Adults, edited by Sharon P. Simson, Laura Wilson, Jared Hermalin, PhD, and Robert E. Hess, PhD* (Vol. 3, No. 1, 1983). *"Highly recommended for professionals and laymen interested in modern viewpoints and techniques for avoiding many physical and mental health problems of the elderly. Written by highly qualified contributors with extensive experience in their respective fields." (The Clinical Gerontologist)*

Strategies for Needs Assessment in Prevention, edited by Alex Zautra, Kenneth Bachrach, and Robert E. Hess, PhD* (Vol. 2, No. 4, 1983). *"An excellent survey on applied techniques for doing needs assessments. . . . It should be on the shelf of anyone involved in prevention." (Journal of Pediatric Psychology)*

Innovations in Prevention, edited by Robert E. Hess, PhD, and Jared Hermalin, PhD* (Vol. 2, No. 3, 1983). *An exciting book that provides invaluable insights on effective prevention programs.*

Rx Television: Enhancing the Preventive Impact of TV, edited by Joyce Sprafkin, Carolyn Swift, PhD, and Robert E. Hess, PhD* (Vol. 2, No. 1/2, 1983). *"The successful interventions reported in this volume make interesting reading on two grounds. First, they show quite clearly how powerful television can be in molding children. Second, they illustrate how this power can be used for good ends." (Contemporary Psychology)*

Early Intervention Programs for Infants, edited by Howard A. Moss, MD, Robert E. Hess, PhD, and Carolyn Swift, PhD* (Vol. 1, No. 4, 1982). *"A useful resource book for those child psychiatrists, paediatricians, and psychologists interested in early intervention and prevention." (The Royal College of Psychiatrists)*

Helping People to Help Themselves: Self-Help and Prevention, edited by Leonard D. Borman, PhD, Leslie E. Borck, PhD, Robert E. Hess, PhD, and Frank L. Pasquale* (Vol. 1, No. 3, 1982). *"A timely volume . . . a mine of information for interested clinicians, and should stimulate those wishing to do systematic research in the self-help area." (The Journal of Nervous and Mental Disease)*

Evaluation and Prevention in Human Services, edited by Jared Hermalin, PhD, and Jonathan A. Morell, PhD* (Vol. 1, No. 1/2, 1982). *Features methods and problems related to the evaluation of prevention programs.*

Index

Printed and bound by CPI Group (UK) Ltd, Croydon, CR0 4YY

17/10/2024

01775686-0001